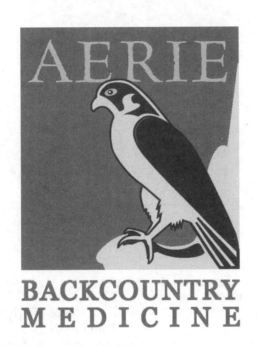

AERIE

BACKCOUNTRY
MEDICINE

WILDERNESS MEDICINE

14th Edition

HW: 5 rights of medication

Wilderness Medicine
14th Edition

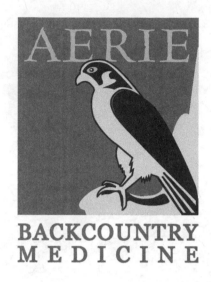

Written By:	Dave McEvoy, MS, Paramedic
	Greg Moore, MD, FACEP, FAWM
	John Bleicher, RN
	Trenton Harper, Paramedic
Contributing Editors to this Edition:	Joe Blattner, MA, AEMT
	Ryan Milling, EMT
	Doug Petch, MS, Paramedic
	Akshay Shah, EMT
Illustrations:	Meg Hanson
	Kathleen Hanson

100 North Ave. West
P.O. Box 8146
Missoula, MT 59807
406.542.9972
info@aeriemed.com
www.aeriemedicine.com

Front and Back Cover Photo: Grey Wolf Peak, Mission Mountains, Montana. Ryan Milling, 2019.

A free downloadable copy of this textbook is available at:
www.aeriemedicine.com/textbook

Acknowledgements:

Aerie would like to recognize the continued efforts of our
instructors for the quality improvement of this Wilderness
Medicine manual. Special distinction goes to Amy Shuler, Eric
Mullen, and Akshay Shah for their time and attention in this
14th edition.

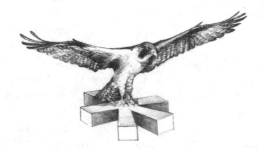

Table of Contents

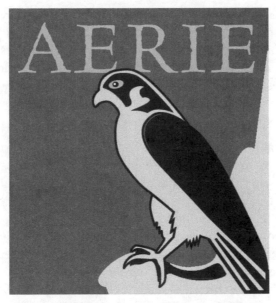

Section One:
Introduction

FA
WFA
WAFA
WFR
EMT
W-EMT

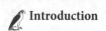

Wilderness Medicine Introduction

Background   *Rule #1 do no harm*

No matter how one defines wilderness medicine, two basic principles should guide the wilderness medicine practitioner:

  1. Nobody dies a preventable death.

  2. Keep simple things simple.

What are preventable deaths in a wilderness setting? Most importantly, they are rescuer deaths: care providers should not perish in the attempt. The greatest disservice a rescuer can provide is the distraction of their own demise. Similarly, uninjured or otherwise healthy people need to remain as such. When dealing with patients, "one and one does not equal two". Two patients are exponentially more difficult to manage than one. Finally, patients die preventable deaths because of failures to correct threats to airway, breathing, circulation, and threats from the environment. In short, avoid preventable deaths by controlling scenes before managing patients and by addressing major threats to life before minor threats to comfort.

What are the simple things that providers should try to keep simple? They include the minor abrasions, mild abdominal discomfort, and blisters that are a part of most adventures lasting longer than a few hours. Anyone who studies disasters will tell you that most occur at the end of a series of minor problems whose significance is underestimated. To a person trained in wilderness medicine, a blister should prompt questions about its cause before actions for its treatment. Are we caring for our feet? Are we moving too quickly for some members of our group? Are we ready to continue the trip? Most importantly, are we paying attention or only lip service to our health? Wilderness medicine practitioners have a unique opportunity to prevent illness and injury. Often, we are not simply responding to calls for help from an anonymous person. Instead, we are there from the beginning, planning the trip, watching the weather, reading the faces of our companions or the state of our own well-being. Our role as a participant in the event, and the opportunities this provides to prevent or at least mitigate the damage, makes the practice of wilderness medicine truly unique.

Manual Layout

Sections of the manual are generally organized as follows:

Epidemiology: Data about the prevalence of injuries or illnesses, with an emphasis on any data that pertains to wilderness and travel medicine as well as urban studies. When available, data will most often be pulled from publications of the Wilderness Medical Society and the US Center for Disease Control, as well as other reliable sources.

Prevention: Key strategies for preventing injuries or illnesses.

Anatomy and Physiology: Drawings, diagrams, and descriptions of the anatomy and physiology relative to the problem.

Signs and Symptoms: Common indications of the specific injury or illness, whether observed by the caregiver (signs) or reported by the patient (symptoms).

Treatment: The steps taken to care for the patient until a higher level of medical care is available.

Critical Thinking: A summation of the most important points covered in the above material, along with suggestions for thinking about these problems in a wilderness setting.

Evacuation Criteria: Considerations for determining how quickly a patient should be transferred to a higher level of medical care.

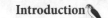

Evidence & Guidelines

Evidence base for the recommendations provided in this manual as well as additional resources:

In cooperation with the Wilderness Medical Society (WMS), and in conjunction with other leading wilderness medical training organizations, Aerie completed a literature review of the efficacy of the recommendations provided in this manual. These are available online at: www.aeriemedicine.com/wms. In addition, the Wilderness Medical Society has separately published Practice Guidelines for many of the injuries and illness discussed in this manual. While intended primarily for physicians, these guidelines form the basis for many of our recommendations. These guidelines are listed here: www.aeriemedicine.com/textbook.

It is critical to recognize that these recommendations are not intended as a substitute for clinical judgment or physician-authorized protocols that are in compliance with all relevant state, national, and where relevant, international guidelines.

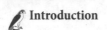

Pertinent Legal Aspects of Wilderness Medicine

Background

The first rule of medicine is unequivocal: do no harm. Clear, yes. Easy, no. We can hurt people while caring for them, by not caring for them, or by providing inappropriate care. In addition, we can be held accountable for any of the above acts if we fail to document accurately.

Wilderness medicine follows most standards established for care in an urban setting: do no harm, provide the care that a reasonable person would provide, and remain within your training. Yet, wilderness medicine differs from urban medicine in a few specific ways. By definition, we provide it when we are hours or days away from care and, as a result, are confronted with the need to treat certain problems on our own rather than waiting for care to arrive. We are also required to make the most difficult decisions of all: whether to evacuate a patient and, if so, by what means.

Law is often based on precedent; has a similar case been tried, and if so, what was the outcome? However, it is important to note that wilderness medicine has very few legal precedents. To date, federal and most state governments have not established a standard of care for a wilderness setting. Instead, individual organizations have developed their own guidelines that begin to define a standard. While these recommendations should fall within state and federal standards of care for a given level of training, they address circumstances not considered in guidelines written for care provided in an urban setting. At times, then, wilderness medicine providers operate on a precarious legal and physical periphery to standard, accepted medical guidelines and practices.

Negligence

Accusations of negligence are, at the core of most charges, leveled against a care provider. To prove negligence, a court must find that all four of the following apply:

1. The care provider had a **duty to act** because they are on duty as emergency personnel, they are a trip leader/guide and one of their party is injured, or they caused the injury or illness.

2. The care provider **breached that duty** by performing or omitting an act that a reasonable person with similar training would or would not have done.

3. The patient suffered **further injuries.**

4. There is proof that those injuries were **caused by the breach of duty** (referred to as "proximal cause").

Standard of Care *look up good sam law for state*

Once the provider does act, they will be judged by:

1. **Reasonable Person Standard** – in comparison to a person of similar training and experience, presented with the identical patient, environment, and resources.

2. **Standards imposed by force of law** – local statutes, ordinances, case law, and administrative orders. Laws may vary from one backcountry setting to another (e.g., different counties, national parks, states, countries, etc.).

3. **Professional or institutional standards** – published recommendations of organizations and societies involved in emergency work and specific rules and procedures of the service for which the provider is a part.

• Always take documentation

Patient Consent

All patients **must consent** to help. This is defined as:

1. **Actual Consent** – An alert and oriented adult may consent after being informed of what the care provider wishes to do. Verbal consent is valid.

2. **Implied Consent** – If the patient is unresponsive or is not mentally competent (see "Patient Competency" below), the law assumes that the patient would give consent.

   - **Minor's Consent** – The right to consent is usually given to the parent or legal guardian. If neither is available after a reasonable effort to locate them, you may treat the patient based upon implied consent.

   - **Mentally Ill or Impaired** – Similar to that of minors. If a guardian is unavailable, treat based upon implied consent. In the case of impairment due to alcohol or drugs, proceed carefully.

Patient Competency

An adult who is alert and oriented to person, place, time, and events is usually considered competent and able to make decisions regarding his or her care.

Patient Refusal of Care

A competent adult has the right to refuse treatment at any time. This is also true of a parent or legal guardian refusing care or treatment for a minor. This refusal must be documented.

Immunities

Because these immunities are variable from state to state, it is important that you familiarize yourself with the specific requirements of the state(s) in which you act.

1. **Good Samaritan Laws** – Every U.S. state has one, but there is variability. Some states grant immunity to those who volunteer to help an injured person at the scene of an accident. These laws do not typically provide immunity to acts of negligence.

2. **Medical Practices Act** – Nearly every state exempts emergency treatment from the licensure requirements for the non-professional.

Abandonment

After initiating care, it can be considered abandonment to either leave a patient or turn the patient over to a person of lesser training. Unless the scene becomes unsafe, the patient is a competent adult and refuses your care, or the patient clearly does not require your level of training.

Summary

You should always strive to provide the best possible care to your patient. It is important to note that you are usually covered by Good Samaritan Laws when you volunteer patient care unless you have a legal duty to act or are employed with the responsibility to provide for the safety and treatment of clients or students. The proper documentation of your patient care is key. Be sure to check laws in your area.

Your best defense is to keep your skills current and to act in a reasonable and prudent manner.

- Never say name over radio

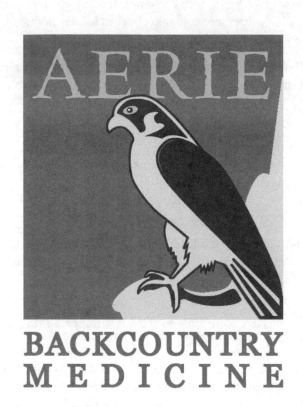

Section Two:
Patient Assessment

Patient Assessment

Background

"Move with intent, look for work."

There is something inherently counter-intuitive about the process of assessment. Obvious injuries are often less important than unseen hazards; the well-being of rescuers takes priority over the health of even the gravely injured. To do this properly, the provider must continuously triage, or sort, scenes and patients, evaluating both with the understanding that threats to life must be managed before threats to limb. The care provider must follow a plan that is both structured and dynamic, anticipating that as scenes and patients change, so too will the priorities of care. No skill is more valuable and difficult to acquire.

Assessment Algorithm

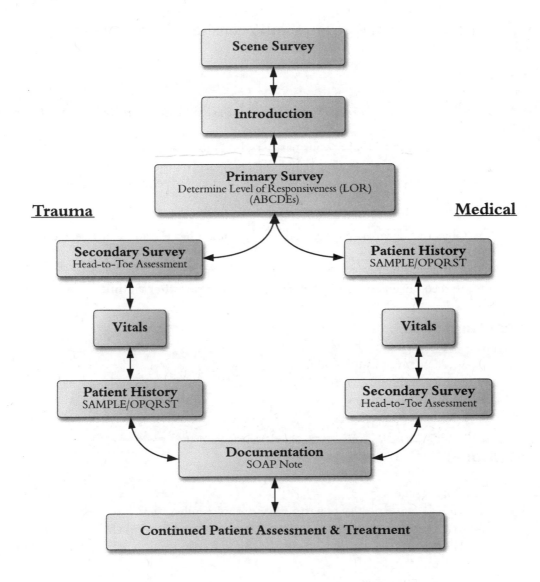

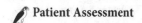

Scene Survey

Background

"Manage scenes before patients."

DEFINITION: During the scene survey, the rescuer evaluates for hazards, tries to understand mechanisms, and begins the process of gathering what is needed to safely and effectively care for the patient. Chaotic scenes encourage hasty surveys, causing rescuers to take unacceptable and unknown risks.

WHEN: The scene survey usually begins with a call for help or a dispatch well before you arrive on scene and continues throughout the scene as you reconsider your needs.

When conducting a scene survey, you should consider the following:

Scene Safety

The greatest disservice a rescuer can provide is the distraction of their own injuries or demise.

- Your safety and that of your partners, bystanders and patients
- Body substance isolation or BSI (e.g., gloves, eye protection, etc.)
- Personal protective equipment or PPE (e.g., closed toed boots, helmet, etc.)
- Time of day
- Weather
- Objective hazards (e.g. rock fall, avalanches, other terrain, violence, etc.)

NOTE: If the situation is unsafe, do not enter it until it is safe to do so, or at least until hazards are recognized and mitigated. **Do not become another victim.**

What Happened

- Mechanism of Injury (MOI)
- Nature of the Illness (NOI)/Chief Complaint (c/c) — *inside body*
- When did it happen?
- Number of patients

Additional Resources

1. More rescuers
2. Knowledge/expertise of partners or group members
3. Extra supplies (i.e., what equipment is needed and how much is currently available?)
4. Alternative evacuation plans (e.g., ground transportation, helicopter evacuation, easier terrain, etc.)
5. Search and rescue
6. Law enforcement

Primary Survey

Background

"Assess for and manage life threats before non-critical injuries and illnesses."

DEFINITION: The purpose of the primary survey is to find all correctable life threats. Nothing about it is academic. The primary survey is conducted with the thought that your patient will die unless you identify and treat their life-threatening problems. The primary survey usually takes about a minute if no threats to life are found.

WHEN: If, at any point, you find a problem during the primary survey, **STOP AND FIX THE PROBLEM**.

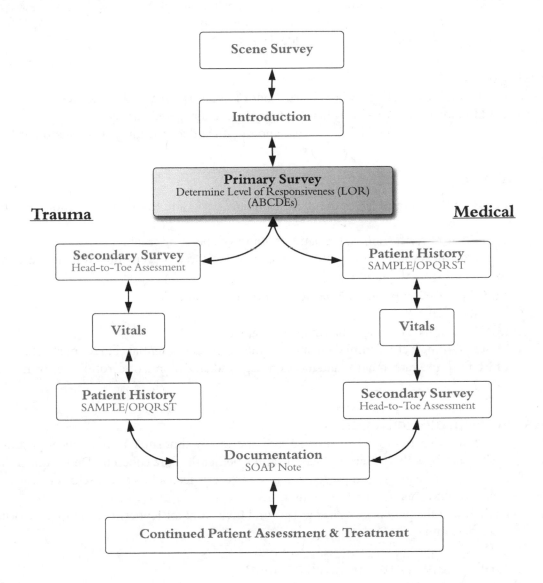

Primary Survey (ABCDEs)

Determine Level of Responsiveness (LOR)

Utilizing the AVPU scale, determine if the patient is **A**lert, responsive to **V**erbal stimulus, responsive to **P**ainful stimulus, or otherwise **U**nresponsive.

LISTEN to their chief complaint, and speech content as indicators of their LOR.

Identify and Control Massive Hemorrhage:

LOOK for signs of life threatening bleeding such as pulsatile or steady bleeding from wounds, blood pooling on ground or saturating clothing, or traumatic amputations. Immediately control life threatening bleeding.

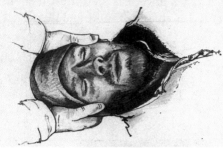

Protect the Spine:

Hold the patient's head stable and minimize movement if you either suspect spinal trauma or you are unsure what caused the injury. *Do not let concern for a possible spinal injury distract you from addressing known life threats.*

"Holding C-Spine"

A Assess Airway:

LOOK for loose teeth or other obstructions or potential obstructions, secretions, or blood.

LISTEN for noise. An airway making noise is an endangered airway.

FEEL for air movement from the nose and mouth and for the integrity of anatomical structures.

B Assess Breathing:

LOOK at the rise and fall of the chest (front and back) and the amount of effort your patient requires to breathe.

LISTEN for breath sounds, the patient's ability to speak, or gasping.

FEEL for chest wall integrity and symmetry of chest wall movement (front and back) and for air movement from the mouth and nose.

• crepitus - bone on bone, crackle sound

C Assess Circulation:

LOOK at skin color, major bleeding, and capillary refill.

LISTEN to their chief complaint and carefully consider potential sources of shock.

FEEL for pulse rate, quality, and location (e.g., radial, femoral, or carotid). Perform a "blood sweep."

D Assess for Neurologic Deficit:

LOOK at the patient's behavior and affect, and/or any abnormal movements or posture.

LISTEN to how the patient is speaking and whether they are coherent. Determine if they are oriented to person, place, time, and events. Ask if they experienced a loss of consciousness and whether they have any abnormal weakness or sensations.

FEEL down the patient's c-spine and around their head for tenderness, physical deformity, or other signs of trauma.

E Protect the patient from the Environment

LOOK at the patient's skin color and their exposure to the environment.

LISTEN to what the patient or bystanders tell you about what happened and how long the patient may have been immobile.

FEEL the temperature of the patient's torso (front and back) and extremities. In general, we must work to keep most patients warm unless they are specifically hot. Any patient that has suffered severe trauma MUST be kept warm, even in the presence of warm ambient temperatures.

Secondary Survey

Background

DEFINITION: The secondary survey, or head-to-toe physical exam, is a systematic, detailed assessment of the whole body that looks for deformities, open wounds, bruising, burns, swelling, or anything else unusual. The rescuer should compare both sides of the body for symmetry, feel for crepitus, tenderness, rigidity, or deformity and ask about pain and smell for unusual odors.

WHEN: This examination is performed only after completion of the primary survey (ABCDEs). If the patient is critically ill or injured, you may not perform a head-to-toe exam because you are busy managing the airway, breathing, or circulation. On the other hand, if you have done a full-body bleed check and an assessment of the major injuries during your primary survey, this may be the third time you physically assess your patient.

WHO: Every patient *deserves* a head-to-toe examination. This is a **systematic, detailed** assessment of the **whole body** that will guide and inform your patient care. Only a problem involving ABCDEs, which must be continuously managed, should prevent you from performing this exam.

DETAILS: It is important that only **one** person performs this exam so that it is systematic and nothing is overlooked. While performing the exam, talk to your patient. Even if a patient is unresponsive, assess for responses to palpation such as wincing, grimacing, or twitching. **To avoid confusing the patient, only one rescuer should talk to the patient at a time.**

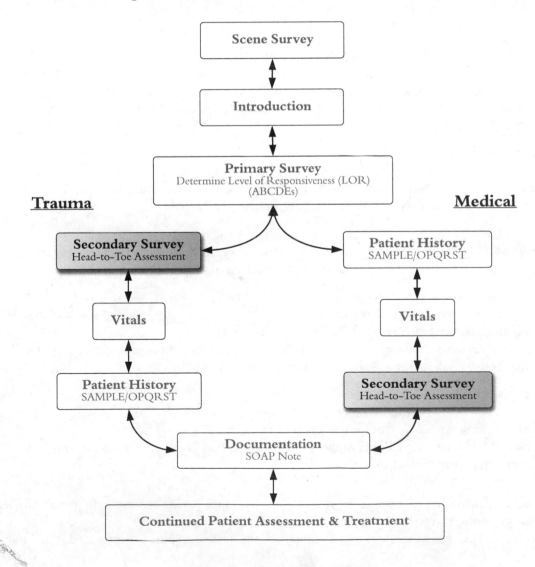

Secondary Survey

Head/Face
- Look into the **mouth** for blood, vomit, loose teeth, or other obstructions.
- Look for blood or cerebrospinal fluid (CSF) draining from **ears** or bruising behind **ears**.
- Look for blood or CSF draining from the **nose**.
- Inspect the **scalp** for stability of the skull bones, bleeding and bruising by removing clothing, and feeling though the hair.
- Evaluate and palpate cautiously for facial fractures.
- Ask the patient if their teeth and jaw feel properly aligned when biting down.
- Check for **pupil** equality and reactivity with a penlight, flashlight, or by shielding the eyes from light with your hand (refer to vital signs).
- Smell the patient's breath for abnormal odors (e.g., alcohol, vomit, etc.).
- Listen for and recognize potential airway swelling dangers.

Cervical Spine (C-Spine)
- Look at all parts of the spine for bruising, swelling, or deformity.
- Palpate down the length of the c-spine while feeling each spinous process and checking for point-tenderness, pain, swelling, crepitus, or deformity.

Neck/Throat
- Examine the neck and throat for any injuries or deformities, or abnormal findings.

Clavicles
- Palpate along each clavicle one at a time, feeling for deformity, tenderness, or pain.

Chest
- Look at the chest wall, front and back, for bruising or wounds.
- Note breathing effort, pain, crepitus, symmetry of chest wall expansion, and/or unusual movement.
- Use both hands to apply resistance to the ribs as the patient takes a deep breath.
- Using the edge of one hand, apply resistance to the sternum and note any pain, crepitus, or instability.

Abdomen (ABD)
- Examine the abdomen for distention (bloating) or bruising.
- Palpate all four quadrants of the abdomen with flat fingers one quadrant at a time. Feel for softness, rigidity, or abnormal masses. Note any tenderness.

Pelvis
- **Gently** press in and then, if no pain or tenderness are present, down on the iliac crest of the pelvis. If any instability, crepitus, or pain is noted **stop** any manipulation immediately.

Legs/Feet
- Look for deformity, discoloration, or obvious injury.
- Palpate the length of each leg for tenderness or deformity.
- Check circulation, sensation, and motion (CSM) on each foot, and compare the strength of both feet simultaneously. Ask about any abnormal weakness or sensations.

Arms/Hands
- Look for deformity, discoloration, or obvious injury.
- Palpate the length of each arm for tenderness or deformity.
- Check CSM on each hand and compare the grip strength of both hands simultaneously. Ask about any abnormal weakness or sensations.

Spine
- Evaluate by palpating each spinous process from the c-spine to the sacrum noting any pain, tenderness, bruising, swelling, crepitus, deformity, or anything else unusual.
- Only log roll as needed maintaining alignment of the neck and spine for suspected spinal injuries.

Aerie Backcountry Medicine © 14th Edition

Vital Signs

Background

DEFINITION: Vital signs include heart rate, blood pressure, respiratory rate, skin, and pupils. Levels of responsiveness are not classically considered a true vital sign, but are included as such. Vital signs are used in conjunction with the physical assessment and patient history to give you an overall assessment of the patient's condition. Vital signs vary by age, physical condition, and level of stress. "Normal" vital signs **DO NOT** guarantee that the patient is doing well, *particularly in young, healthy patients.*

Baseline Vitals are taken to provide a reading of the patient's initial condition against which future sets are compared. These are the first vitals recorded on a patient.

Vital Sign Trends are consecutive and numerous sets of recorded vital signs that, in combination with your ongoing assessment, will help you figure out how well your patient is doing. Most importantly, changes and trends in a person's vital signs are more useful than an isolated set of vitals because they tell you something about how the patient's injury or illness is progressing.

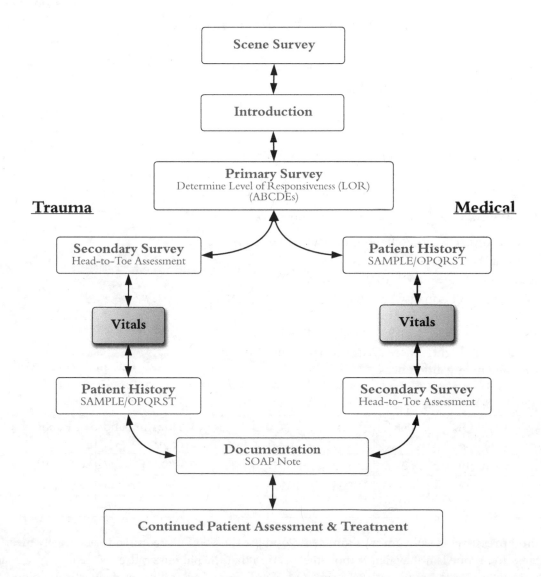

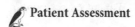

Vital Signs

1. Level of Responsiveness (LOR)

w o r s e n i n g ↓

AVPU Scale:

	1	2	3	4
Alert and Oriented - The patient is oriented to	**Person**	**Place**	**Time**	**Event**

A&O X 4: ████████████████████████

A&O X 3: ███████████████████

A&O X 2: ████████████

A&O X 1: ███

Responsive to Verbal stimulus – Patient only follows commands (e.g., "Blink your eyes").

Responsive to Painful stimulus – Patient only responds to sternum rub or skin pinch.

Unresponsive – Patient does not noticeably respond to any stimulus.

2. Heart Rate (HR) – Check the pulse for 30 seconds and multiply by 2.

RATE: 60 – 100 beats per minute is a normal range for an adult at rest.

RHYTHM: Note whether the beats are regular or irregular.

QUALITY: Note the location taken (radial, femoral, carotid) and its strength (weak, strong, thready).

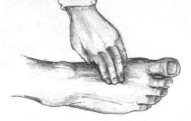

Assessing a pedal pulse

3. Respiratory Rate (RR) – Watch the chest rise for 30 seconds and multiply by 2.

RATE: 12 – 20 breaths per minute in adults is a normal range.

RHYTHM: Regular or Irregular.

QUALITY: Unlabored or Labored.

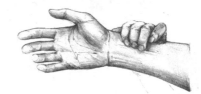

Assessing a radial pulse

4. Skin – Assess the Skin's Color, Temperature, and Moisture (SCTM).

COLOR: Look at non-pigmented areas such as fingernails, mucous membranes inside mouth, and conjunctiva of the eyes. Pink (normal), Pale, Flushed, Cyanotic (bluish).

TEMPERATURE: Hot, Cold, or Warm (normal).

MOISTURE: Clammy/Diaphoretic (sweaty) or Dry (normal).

5. Pupils – Check for equality between the right and left pupils and check for reactivity to light.

Normal pupils are PERRL: Pupils are Equal, Round, and Reactive to Light. These are normal findings. Note and document any differences.

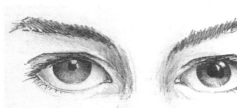

Unequal and Irregular Pupil

Example:

TIME	LOR	RR	HR	SCTM	BP or pulse location and strength	Pupils
1635	A&Ox3	22	110	PWD	130/90	PERRL
1640	A&Ox3	20	106	PWD	126/80	PERRL
1645						

A note about blood pressure: A sphygmomanometer (blood pressure cuff) is required to accurately measure a patient's blood pressure. If one is not available, note the location that the patient's pulse was felt - typically at either the radial or carotid artery - and its strength. A strong radial pulse is a good indicator of a perfusing blood pressure.

Patient History (SAMPLE/OPQRST)

Background

DEFINITION: Taking a patient history involves asking questions that will help the patient elaborate on a specific problem, as well as help you obtain clues as to what else might be complicating the situation.

DETAILS: As with the physical exam, the patient history should be **systematic** and **thorough**. The following acronym and mnemonic will guide you to the more important questions to ask. Maintaining a high **index of suspicion** for underlying injuries based on your assessment, gut instincts, and mechanisms of injury should guide your questioning in order to gain more insight about the patient's condition.

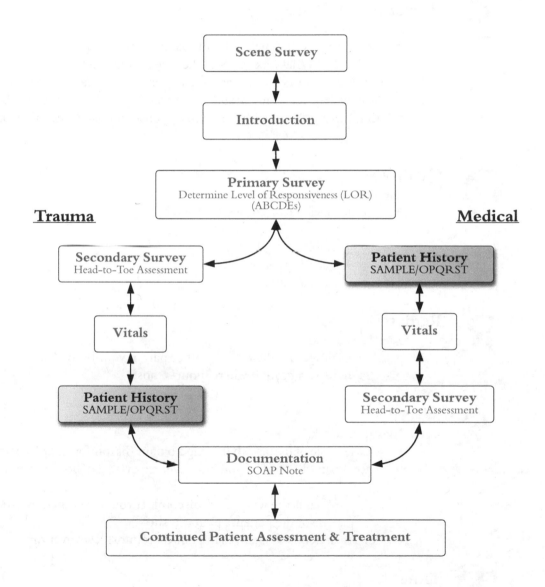

Patient History (SAMPLE/OPQRST)

S **Signs and Symptoms (S/S)**
Signs are what you find during your physical assessment (objective information); whereas, *symptoms* are complaints the patient tells you (subjective information). The main problem may also be stated as the "**Chief Complaint**" (documented c/c).

(**OPQRST**) Elaborate on the chief complaint or symptoms with these questions:

O **Onset**
Questions to ask:
- "Did the pain come on gradually or suddenly?"
  - Did it begin with an event, such as trauma, eating meals, stress, etc.?

P **Provokes or Palliates**
Questions to ask:
- Provoke – "What makes the problem worse?"
- Palliate – "What relieves or makes the problem better?"

NOTE: A person in pain will assume the position of least discomfort, so pay attention to how they are sitting, standing, or walking, and see if they are bracing or self-splinting (i.e., holding their arm tightly against their side when they breathe).

Q **Quality**
Questions to ask:
- "What does the discomfort feel like?"
  - Sharp/ dull
  - Stabbing/ throbbing
  - Squeezing/ pressure
  - Itching/ burning

R **Radiates**
Questions to ask:
- "Does the pain radiate to any other part of your body?"
- "Is there pain beyond where it hurts most?"

S **Severity**
Questions to ask:
- "On a scale of 0-10, with 0 being no pain/discomfort and 10 being the worst pain/discomfort you have ever experienced, how do you rate this pain?"
  - "What is the worst pain/discomfort you have experienced?" (to get a sense of the patient's pain threshold)

NOTE: Track trends or changes in pain/discomfort level over time.

T **Time**
Questions to ask:
- "When did this first occur?"
- "What else was happening then?"

A Allergies

Ask about:
- Foods
- Medications
- Animals (primarily insects)
- Plants
- Other

M Medications

Questions to ask:
- What medications are you currently taking?
  - Name of medication
  - How often it is taken (and has there been any recent changes to frequency)?
  - How much is taken (and has there been any recent changes to dosages)?
  - For which medical condition it is taken?
- Any medications prescribed but not taken regularly?
  - Include over-the-counter (OTC), alternative, or recreational medications.
- Any medications recently discontinued or has there been any recent changes to dosages?

P Past Pertinent Medical History (PMH)

Questions to ask, if relevant:
- Have you experienced this problem before?
  - If so, what was the diagnosis?
  - What is different about this time?
- Is there a family history of this problem?
- Have you been hospitalized for this condition or for anything else lately?
- Is there a medical history of other problems?
  - Diabetes
  - Lung problems
  - Mental illness, or depression, particularly any requiring hospitalization or medication
- Is there a possibility of pregnancy?

L Last Oral Intake and Output

Questions to ask:
- What have you had to eat in the last 24 hours?
  - How much?
  - Appetite?
- What liquid did you drink in the last 24 hours?
  - How much?
  - Thirst?
- Can you describe the color and quantity of stool and urine?
  - What is normal output and is this abnormal?
  - Was there pain with urination or defecation?
  - Specifically, any diarrhea?

E Events Leading up to this Problem

Questions to ask:
- What *exactly* happened?
- What were you doing at the time the problem occurred?
- What were the events of the past 24 hours?
- Was anyone with the patient or a witness to the events?

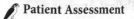

Written and Verbal Patient Reports (SOAP note/ACT-MIST report)

Background

Written and verbal reports are important components of patient care. They remind you of what to look for and what to ask. In addition, written and verbal reports are essential for good communication and the continuity of care. The quality of your assessment and patient care are reflected in these reports as they will improve the next caregiver's ability to treat the patient thoroughly and correctly. Documented reports also have significant legal importance. Take time preparing them. Only factual information should be included. It is crucial that you write legibly and speak clearly.

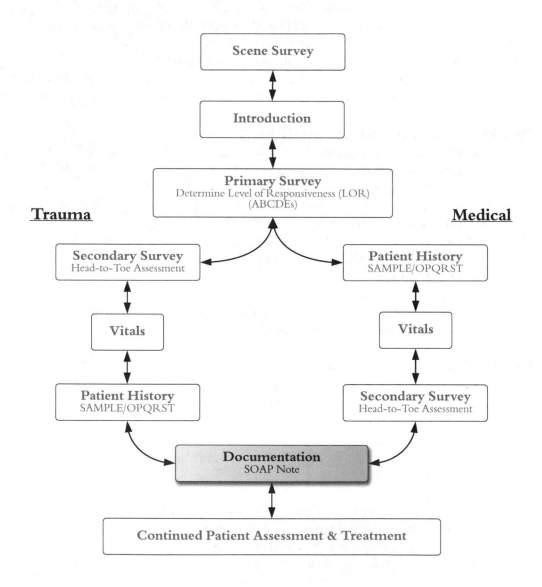

Verbal Patient Reports (ACT-MIST report)

Example:

ACT-MIST Report
Report <u>A</u>ge, <u>C</u>hief Complaint, <u>T</u>ime of Incident, <u>M</u>echanism of Injury, <u>I</u>njuries found, Vital <u>S</u>igns, <u>T</u>reatment When you hand-off your patient to another care provider, give a succinct, pertinent report covering: <u>A</u>ge <u>C</u>hief Complaint <u>T</u>ime of Incident <u>M</u>echanism of Injury/Nature of Illness <u>I</u>njuries Found/Pertinent Physical Findings Vital <u>S</u>igns <u>T</u>reatment

ACT-MIST Report
• This is a 27 year-old with a chief complaint of 10 out of 10 pain to the right lower leg. • At 1330 today the pt fell approximately 20 feet down a rocky hillside. They deny a loss of consciousness before or after event. • Pt has bruising and deformity to the right anterior lower leg. There is a palpable pedal pulse and intact sensation distally with limited ankle movement due to pain. Physical exam is otherwise unremarkable. • Vital signs taken at 1345: A&Ox4, HR 98; RR 22; skin is pink, warm and dry; and pupils are PERRL. • We have splinted and elevated the injured leg. We are continuing to monitor the patient. • We are currently 2 miles up Trout Creek Trail and are requesting assistance with evacuation.

Written Report (SOAP Note)

SOAP NOTE

<u>S</u>ubjective, <u>O</u>bjective, <u>A</u>ssessment, <u>P</u>lan
 	
<u>S</u>ubjective –What your patient or bystanders tell you: -Age   -Chief Complaint (c/c)
        -MOI   -AMPLE
        -OPQRST
 	
<u>O</u>bjective - What you find:
        -ABCDEs   -Head-to-Toe
        -Vital signs
 	
<u>A</u>ssessment - The injuries or illnesses you identified or suspected underlying injuries or illnesses
 	
<u>P</u>lan - What you have done and plan to do for your patient, including evacuation plans, backup plans, and injury treatments

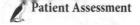

SOAP Note - Front

Aerie Backcountry Medicine
Wilderness Incident SOAP Notes

SUBJECTIVE

Patient's name:	Age_____ Weight _____ lb DOB_____
Location: Lat: Long:	MOI:

Environment: Fall?   Distance?   Helmet?   MVC?   Speed?   Seat Belt?

Other Patients: Y / N   How Many?

SUBJECTIVE: Patient History

Chief Complaint (S/S):

O:	A:
P:	M:
Q:	P:
R:	L:
S:	E:
T:	

OBJECTIVE: Patient Physical Exam

A:	Clear_____ Obstructed_____	**ABD:**	Pain_____	Soft_____
B:	Labored_____ Non-Labored_____		Tender____	Rigid_____
C:	Radial_____ Carotid_____	**Back:**	Pain_____	Deformity____
	Pulse Strong_____ Weak_____		Tender____	
	Major Bleeds_____ Bruising_____	**Pelvis:**	Stable_____	Unstable_____
D:			Tender____	Rigid_____
E:		**Extremities:** (CSM)		
Head:		RA:	LA:	
Neck/Spine:	Tender____ Pain____ Deformity____			
Chest:	Tender_____ Pain_____	RL:	LL:	
	Crepitus_____ Equal Expansion____			

VITAL SIGNS:

Time	LOR	RR	HR	SCTM	BP	Pupils

SOAP Note - Back

Aerie Backcountry Medicine
Wilderness Incident SOAP Notes

ASSESSMENT of Situation and Plan of Treatment

Injury List	Potential Problems

PLAN of Action

Urgency: Critical_____ Stable_____ Minor_____

Patient: Ambulatory_____ Litter Carry_____ Spinal Motion Restriction _____

Injury/illness:	Action Taken:	Planned Treatment:

Evacuation Plan (including back-up plan):

Notes

Aerie Backcountry Medicine © 14th Edition

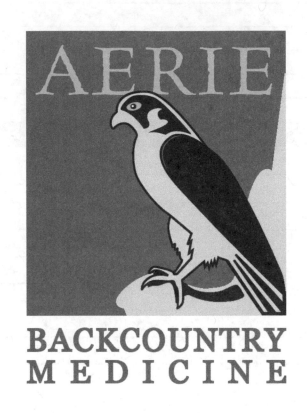

Section Three:
Basics of Patient Management

Airway Management

Background

It is the task of the respiratory system to deliver oxygen and remove carbon dioxide from the blood. For this to occur, the patient must have an unobstructed airway.

DEFINITION:

> **Obstructions** - The most common airway obstruction in the unresponsive **adult** patient is the **tongue**. _Snoring is a very ominous sound._
>
> Blood, vomit, excessive saliva or other foreign objects, broken teeth, food, and gum must all be removed from the mouth or nose.

WHEN: After performing the scene size-up and in the absence of life-threatening bleeding, **airway management is the first priority** in the care of the patient.

WHO: A patient without a patent airway will soon die. Obstructed airways are often overlooked!

DETAILS: When managing a patient's airway, keep the following goals in mind:

1. Examine the mouth and throat for obstructions.
2. Open the airway by moving the tongue away from the back of the throat.
3. Ensure that the c-spine is protected from further injury.
4. Administer artificial respirations (rescue breaths).
5. Prevent or reduce the potential for aspiration of foreign contents into the lungs.

NOTE: If the equipment is available, suctioning the airway may be necessary.

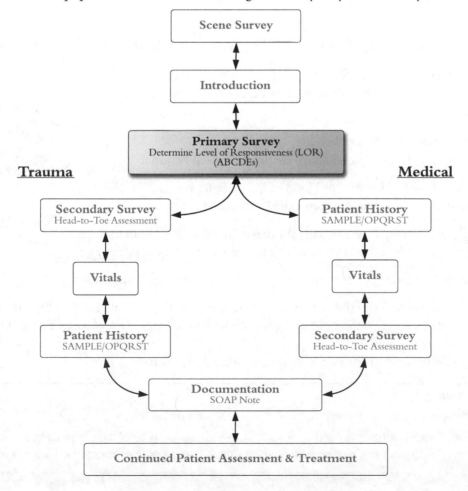

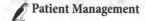
Airway Maneuvers

Airway Techniques for a <u>SNORING PATIENT</u> (tongue obstruction)

1. Head Tilt-Chin Lift

- Appropriate only for the **non-trauma**, unresponsive patient.
- Provides room for rescue breaths.
- Lifts tongue off the back of the throat which lifts the epiglottis from the opening to the trachea.
- Appropriate for **snoring** (tongue), but not gurgling (fluid) patients.
- Will move the c-spine, but may be necessary for adequate breathing or rescue breathing.

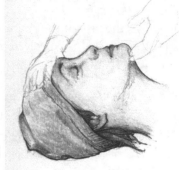

Head Tilt-Chin Lift

2. Jaw-Thrust

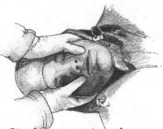

Single-rescuer jaw thrust

Push straight down on the cheekbone and pull straight up at the corner of the jaw.
Do not rotate the head.

- Appropriate for an unresponsive patient with a **potential c-spine injury.**
- Appropriate for **snoring,** but not gurgling patients.
- Lifts the tongue from the back of the throat.
- Allows a full view of the mouth and throat.
- Does not move the c-spine.
- Allows the rescuer room to administer artificial breaths.
- Is very tiring and difficult to maintain during long-term care and potentially impossible to maintain during evacuation.

NOTE: If patient breathing or rescue breaths are ineffective with the jaw-thrust, consider the head tilt-chin lift technique.

Airway Techniques for a <u>GURGLING PATIENT</u> or other partial obstructions

1. **Turn head and gutter or finger sweep**
   - Appropriate only when there is **no trauma** or suspicion of spinal injury.

2. **Log roll and gutter or finger sweep**
   - Appropriate for any patient with **suspected spinal trauma.**

Guttering: Used for fluid, vomit or blood in the patient's mouth. Use the following techniques if the patient is **gurgling** rather than snoring.

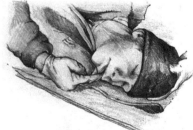

"Guttering" a patient's airway

- Using one finger, draw the patient's cheek down to allow fluid to drain.
- In the case of blood and vomit, this may have to be done repeatedly.

Finger Sweep: Used for objects such as food, chewing gum, teeth, and chewing tobacco.

- If you cannot identify the potential obstruction, turn the patient's head or log roll the patient onto one side and **sweep** the debris out of the mouth with your finger (**watch your fingers**) to clear a potential airway obstruction.
- Do not attempt a finger sweep if you can not see the obstruction.

Evacuation Criteria

Rapidly evacuate any patient who is unable to maintain their own airway.

NOTE: The best way to maintain a clear airway during evacuation is to place the patient on one side. This can be challenging if spinal motion restriction is a priority. One rescuer **must** monitor the patient's airway at all times.

Backcountry CPR

Deciding when not to initiate CPR

Use these criteria with caution and in conjunction with other criteria, ABCDEs, and common sense.

1. Injuries that are incompatible with life such as decapitation or complete evisceration.
2. **Rigor Mortis** – Stiffening of the body after death. It usually begins 1-2 hours after death, initially most obvious in loose joints such as the jaw (you'll notice because you won't be able to do a jaw-thrust), fingers, toes, wrists, and neck.
3. **Dependent Lividity** – Pooling of dark blood (appears black) in dependent areas of the body (e.g., back and buttocks if patient is supine).
4. **Obvious decomposition** – Distinct odor, rotting flesh.
5. Cool temperature without exposure to cold.

Exceptions to the above criteria

1. **Hypothermia** – No issues of CPR are more controversial than either starting or stopping CPR with a hypothermic patient. Some states, such as Alaska, have developed their own protocols to guide the rescuer. Most guidelines are based on two critical concepts. First, a very cold but still-beating heart can, ironically, be *stopped* by the trauma of CPR itself. Therefore, you must have some heightened level of confidence that your patient is truly dead before beginning compressions. Second, hypothermia does confer some protection to a cold heart, extending the window for successfully resuscitating a patient. As a result, once begun, CPR on a hypothermic patient is sometimes continued for a longer period than on a person with a normal body temperature. In either case, it is critical for rescuers to recognize that CPR alone rarely revives a pulseless heart. Prolonged CPR in the backcountry, therefore, is typically a futile exercise.
2. **Hypoxia** – People who are severely oxygen-deprived (hypoxic) will turn dark blue. Oxygenation of these patients may improve their condition.
3. Patients with **infections**, as in gangrene resulting from frostbite, may have severely decomposed flesh.

NOTE: Care should be initiated on all patients that you deem to have a chance of survival. However, in non-hypothermic patients without a pulse, even with effective CPR, irreversible brain damage usually occurs within 6-10 minutes.

NOTE: **Pre-morbid Status** – Odds of successful resuscitation are best if patient is young and healthy before injury or illness.

Deciding when to STOP CPR

In most cases, stopping CPR means you are recognizing that resuscitation efforts are futile or, in rare circumstances, your patient recovered. These times are fortunately few and rare, yet conceptually and emotionally difficult for any rescuer. You may need to make the decision to stop CPR when:

1. **Numerous patients** are involved and your efforts are needed for those patients with a chance of survival.
2. It is **unsafe** for you to attempt a rescue – consider the effects of exhausting your crew and other environmental hazards.
3. The patient has injuries or signs that are **incompatible with life** (rigor mortis, dependent lividity, etc.).
4. You become too **exhausted** to continue.
5. You are **relieved by others** with equal or greater medical training.
6. The patient **regains a pulse** (or other signs of circulation) and does not require continued chest compressions. Patients with a Return Of Spontaneous Circulation (ROSC) often experience subsequent episode(s) of cardiac arrest; continuous monitoring of circulation is imperative.
7. You perform CPR for ½ hour, the patient is not hypothermic, and Advanced Life Support (ALS) is more than an hour away.

- Child CPR: 2m at 30:2 then call 911 start breaths asap for kids

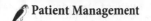

Stress Injuries and Psychological First Aid

Background

"Between stimulus and response there is a space. In that space is our power to choose our response. In our response lies our growth and freedom" - Viktor Frankl

DEFINITIONS:

Stress Reaction - Occurring during an event, a normal stress reaction includes a physiological response to physical and/or psychological stress or trauma from the sympathetic nervous system, a branch of the autonomic nervous system (the branch of the nervous system not under conscious control). This survival reaction by the sympathetic nervous system is often referred to as the "fight or flight" response and is responsible for the spectrum of signs we might encounter in both patients and rescuers. These include changes in vital signs such as elevated heart and respiratory rate, elevated blood pressure, pale skin, sweating, dilated pupils, and changes in cognitive abilities. Other potential effects include tunnel vision (narrowing of the visual field), auditory exclusion (not registering sounds), loss of fine and complex motor skills, tremors, and dissociation (detachment from physical and emotional reality).

Stress Injury - A term that refers to the spectrum of potential psychological effects from exposure to physically or emotionally traumatic events. Post Traumatic Stress Disorder (PTSD) is one long-term example of stress injury.

Psychological First Aid (PFA) - First developed to assist survivors of terrorism and natural disasters, the concepts of PFA have been adopted for use in other emergency scenarios and are particularly relevant to the stressors experienced by both patients and rescuers during wilderness emergencies. The intent of PFA is to provide early intervention for those experiencing a stress reaction to assist with immediate and long term coping mechanisms and ultimately decrease the incidents of stress injury to patients and providers.

WHEN: The concepts of PFA can be implemented throughout an actual or perceived emergency and after the emergency is resolved.

WHO: Any patient and/or provider involved in traumatic or stressful event(s), including one's self. It is important to note that one need not have experienced an injury to experience acute stress. A participant of a near-miss, an event in which injury or harm may have occurred but was avoided, may still experience a stress reaction and can benefit from PFA.

DETAILS: Patients, bystanders, and care providers involved in an emergency may have reactions that include anxiety, fear, grief, guilt, confusion, hopelessness, shame, sleeplessness, and disillusionment. Your interaction with them may help alleviate these reactions and promote long term recovery.

When faced with an overwhelmingly stressful incident, the brain enters survival mode. This heightened level of stress can cause psychological injury if the brain does not revert back to a sense of feeling safe. Over time, repetition of this pattern can cause the brain to avoid similar situations in an attempt to survive. This can look like a lack of interest in participating in a rescue after a particularly hard incident where a responder felt helpless or out of control. Psychological First Aid provides objective strategies for the immediate care of our emotional and psychological wellbeing, which may help prevent the development of stress injury.

Psychological First Aid

Tools for helping patients and care providers during stressful events

1. **Promote a sense of safety-** When possible, move patients to a safe place and promote an awareness of safety with clear and accurate communication. Otherwise, take deliberate actions to mitigate safety concerns and diminish the sense of chaos that often accompanies emergencies.

2. **Promote calming-** Take deliberate steps to calm yourself before and during an emergency. Communicate "calm" to your patient with your deliberate actions, words, and tone; be friendly and compassionate. Coach your patient to take deep breaths as appropriate to the situation and their condition.

3. **Promote a sense of self and collective efficacy-** To the extent possible, include the patient in their own care and the decision making. When possible, include other party members in the process as well.

4. **Promote connectedness-** Promote a sense of connection between the patient, yourself, and other members of the party. Ask the patient what they would like to be called and use it regularly. When possible help those in need contact friends or loved ones.

5. **Promote hope-** Cultivate and maintain the belief that things will get better. Communicate to your patient the specific tangible actions you have taken to improve the situation. Remind your patient that more help is on the way, if you know that to be true.

Improving Rescuer Performance Under Stress

Techniques for maintaining performance during an emergency

Adapted from *Psychological Skills to Improve Emergency Care Providers' Performance Under Stress*, Lauria et al.

1. **Breathe**: Use performance-enhancing breathing. Prior to, during, and between stressful events utilize deep, slow breathing with an emphasis on prolonged inhalation through the nose, pausing before exhalation, then a prolonged exhalation through the mouth. This can counteract the negative effects of the sympathetic nervous system response.

2. **Talk**: Use positive self talk. Develop a habit of positive internal dialogue to guide confident performance. Positive self talk can be instructional, motivational, mood-related, and self-affirmative, such as "Lift the jaw forward", "I can do this", or "I am well-trained".
   a. Keep phrases short and specific.
   b. Use first person and present tense.
   c. The phrases should be positive as opposed to negative.
   d. When you recite a phrase to yourself, say it with intention.
   e. Speak kindly to yourself.
   f. Repeat phrases often.

3. **See**: Use visualization exercises, imagery, and mental practice. Visualize the specific skill, task, or scenario you are preparing to perform. This could be performing an airway maneuver, applying a splint, or the steps of a patient assessment.

4. **Focus**: Develop and use a focus word or phrase. Under the stress of a wilderness emergency, it is possible to become mentally overwhelmed by the complexity of the situation. Utilize a practiced word such as "focus" or "breathe", or a phrase such as "slow is smooth, smooth is fast" to focus the mind on the task at hand or to maintain situational awareness.

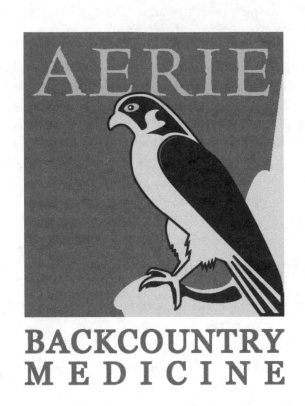

Section Four:
Traumatic Emergencies

Bleeding and Shock   • Flat, dry, warm

Background

The circulatory system delivers oxygen and nutrients while removing waste products, such as carbon dioxide, from the cells. Perfusion refers to this delivery of oxygen and glucose to the cells and removal of carbon dioxide, which is generally required by the cells to produce energy and function normally. Requirements for perfusion of the body's tissues include: adequate oxygenation of the blood via the respiratory system (a patent airway and adequate breathing), adequate cardiac output (the heart's ability to pump blood), adequate blood volume, and adequate blood pressure.

DEFINITION: Shock is defined as inadequate tissue perfusion, resulting in cellular and organ dysfunction. Inadequate perfusion causes a shift from aerobic to anaerobic metabolism, decreasing energy production and increasing acid build-up in the body. The decrease in energy production reduces body temperature and leads to hypothermia. The acidotic state decreases the body's ability to form and maintain clots, called coagulopathy. Hypothermia also decreases the body's ability to form and maintain clots, thus exacerbating coagulopathy. The self perpetuating triad of acidosis, coagulopathy, and hypothermia is referred to as "the lethal triad".

ANATOMY AND PHYSIOLOGY: There are many causes of shock. Most relate to three main types:

- **Hypovolemic Shock:** Problems with the fluid (blood volume)

- **Cardiogenic Shock:** Problems with the pump (cardiac function)

- **Distributive/ Vasogenic Shock:** Problems with the vessels (vascular dilation and permeability)
  - ‣ Anaphylaxis – allergies
  - ‣ Sepsis – infection
  - ‣ Psychogenic – stress, fear, pain
  - ‣ Neurogenic – spinal cord injury

DETAILS: In the wilderness setting, the most prevalent form of shock is **hypovolemic shock**. Common causes of hypovolemic shock include hemorrhage (bleeding), which can be obvious (external) or subtle (internal). Hypovolemic shock can occur without hemorrhage when the body loses fluid via other means such as dehydration (often from vomiting and/or diarrhea) or burns.

Signs & Symptoms of Hypovolemic Shock

The body responds to shock via stimulation of the sympathetic nervous system and by releasing hormones such as epinephrine and norepinephrine. This "fight or flight" response allows the body to **compensate** for the circulatory deficiency and causes many of the signs and symptoms seen in shock. Shock is progressive. As the body gradually loses the ability to **compensate** for the circulatory deficiency, the patient presents with worsening signs and symptoms, eventually resulting in death.

Typical Vital Signs of Compensatory Shock:

1. LOR: Anxiety, restlessness progressing to confusion and unresponsiveness

2. HR: Rapid distal pulses becoming progressively weaker

3. RR: Rapid, shallow, or deep

4. Skin: Pale (possibly cyanotic), cool, clammy, or sweaty; delayed capillary refill

5. Pupils: Dilated and sluggish

6. Additional S/S: dizziness or fainting (especially when upright), weakness, fatigue, thirst, decreased urine output, nausea, vomiting

NOTE: A drop in blood pressure (BP) is the hallmark of a body no longer able to compensate for circulatory collapse. Without a BP cuff, you will notice this with a loss of distal pulses and a significant drop in level of responsiveness.

Treatment for Shock

1. ABCDEs – Immediately identify and control any **massive external hemorrhage**.

    A: Open and maintain the **airway**.

    B: Assist **ventilations**, if necessary; provide supplemental oxygen, if available.

    C: Lay the patient flat to assist **circulation** to the brain and other vital organs. Treat specific injuries that may contribute to further blood loss (e.g., splint fractures, apply pelvic wrap).

    D: Monitor patient's LOR as an indicator of perfusion status.

    E: **Keep the patient warm**. Protect the patient from the **environment** by placing them in a hypothermia wrap.

2. **Comfort, Calm, and Reassure the Patient** – When caring for your patient, be sincere, compassionate, and act confidently. Don't offer obviously false hope; rather, reassure the patient that you are going to help them.

3. **Fluid** – While the patient is sitting upright, you can give small sips of water at regular intervals only if you are providing long-term care and the patient can tolerate it. Are they able to manage their own airway and water does not cause nausea?

4. **Ongoing Assessment** – Because shock is progressive, systematically reassess the patient and carefully evaluate trends in vitals signs.

External Bleeding

Background

• Artial bleed bright red, spurting
• vanus bleed dark red, pooling

Bleeding/hemorrhage is a major cause of potentially preventable deaths, both on the battlefield and in the civilian setting. Much research and real-world experience, primarily from military forces guided by the Committee for Tactical Combat Casualty Care (CoTCCC), has led to a strong evidence base for hemorrhage control techniques that are now standards of care within the civilian sector. Life-threatening bleeding should be addressed early in the primary assessment. A patient with an uncontrolled arterial bleed can die from exsanguination (i.e., 'bleeding out') within minutes. It is worth noting that not all bleeding is life-threatening.

DEFINITION: Life-threatening bleeding and other wounds requiring tourniquet application or other aggressive means of hemorrhage control can be identified by pulsating or steady bleeding, blood pooling on the ground or saturating overlying clothing, standard bandaging that is ineffective and steadily saturated with blood, complete or partial amputations, or prior bleeding from a wound in a patient that is now in shock.

Treatment

1. **Body Substance Isolation (BSI)** – Use protective gloves, eyewear, and clothing as necessary.

2. Have the patient sit or **lay down**.

3. **ABCDEs** – Quickly identify open wounds and **note the severity of bleeding**. Control any life-threatening external hemorrhage immediately before addressing airway or breathing problems.

4. Treat for **shock**, maintain warmth and protect from environment with hypowrap.

5. **Splint injured extremities** to immobilize and minimize blood flow.

Bleeding Control

1. **Direct Pressure**: Use a gloved hand to apply pressure directly onto the bleeding site. For heavy bleeds you may need to apply a significant amount of pressure using one or both hands, often enough to cause pain. You may ask the patient to hold the pressure, if they are able to do so, while you collect your bleeding control supplies. If direct pressure easily controls the bleeding maintain the pressure manually or with a less-aggressive pressure dressing.

    • **If direct pressure is not effective, immediately apply a tourniquet.**

2. **Wound Packing and Pressure Dressing:** Use when direct pressure is effective but difficult to maintain, a tourniquet is not available, or a tourniquet must be transitioned due to extended patient care times exceeding 2 hours from time of tourniquet application.

   1. Expose the wound while maintaining direct pressure.

   2. Wipe away any pooled blood and tightly pack roll gauze or similar material into the wound. Maintain continuous pressure during your efforts.

   3. Focus initial packing efforts on any sites of obvious pulsating or flowing blood.

   4. Pack the wound cavity tightly with gauze until no further gauze can be pushed into the wound.

   5. Mound additional gauze over the site.

   6. Application of pressure via a bandage will preferentially push pressure into the wound.

      • If using hemostatic impregnated gauze, hold manual direct pressure for 3 minutes before applying a pressure dressing.

      • For minor wounds that do not require aggressive packing, apply additional pressure with a roll gauze.

   7. If bleeding continues, or has already required aggressive packing, apply a stretch bandage (ACE™ wrap, Coban™, or manufactured trauma dressing) over and around the site removing the stretch with each wrap until bleeding is obviously controlled. Secure the outer bandage and note the time of application.

   • **If the above efforts fail, immediately apply/reapply a tourniquet.**

Tourniquet Use

In the presence of life-threatening bleeding a tourniquet should be applied. A properly-applied tourniquet will hurt.

1. Identify all wounds to the involved extremity.
2. Apply the tourniquet 2-3 inches proximal to the injury. Do not apply directly over joints. Avoid application immediately above the knee joint.
3. If unable to determine the full extent of injuries, apply "high and tight" to the most proximal aspect of the extremity.
4. Remove any slack from the device before turning the windlass.
5. Turn the windlass, tightening the tourniquet until bleeding stops and distal pulses are lost.
6. Do not apply a partial tourniquet. This blocks venous return but does not completely occlude arterial blood flow to the extremity. This can result in damage to the extremity.
7. Properly secure the tourniquet.
8. Mark the time of application.
   • If the first properly-applied tourniquet is not effective, a second tourniquet should be applied immediately above (or proximal to) the first tourniquet.

NOTE: Effective improvised tourniquets are difficult to construct and are statistically not as effective as manufactured tourniquets; if the need for a tourniquet is anticipated, carry a manufactured device recommended by the CoTCCC.

Common Tourniquet Application Mistakes

1. Not using one when indicated
2. Waiting too long to apply
3. Not pulling the slack out before turning windlass (too loose)
4. Using tourniquet for minor bleeding
5. Too proximal of placement when wound is clearly visible distally
6. Not removing or transitioning to a pressure dressing during extended patient care
7. Taking it off when it should not be removed (when patient is in shock or during short transport times)
8. Not applying tight enough (allowing for arterial blood flow while occluding venous return)
9. Not using a second tourniquet when indicated
10. Periodically loosening the tourniquet

Hemorrhage Control for Significant Bleeding

Identify wounds with significant bleeding – pulsating/steady bleeding, pooling or saturating clothing, standard bandaging ineffective/steadily saturated, complete or partial amputations, prior significant bleeding with patient now in shock

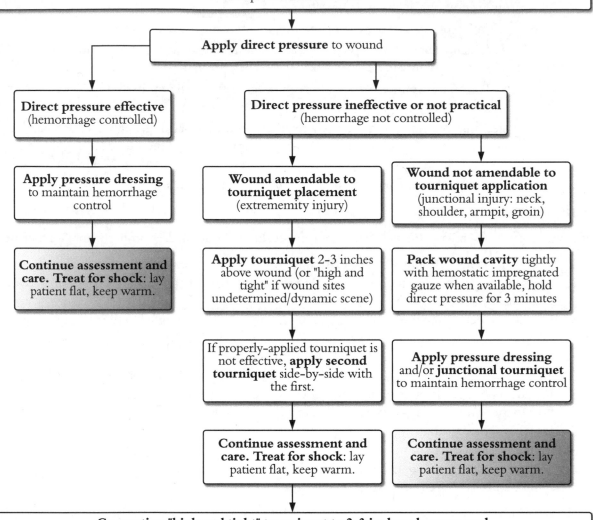

Apply direct pressure to wound

Direct pressure effective
(hemorrhage controlled)

Direct pressure ineffective or not practical
(hemorrhage not controlled)

Apply pressure dressing to maintain hemorrhage control

Wound amendable to tourniquet placement (extrememity injury)

Wound not amendable to tourniquet application (junctional injury: neck, shoulder, armpit, groin)

Continue assessment and care. Treat for shock: lay patient flat, keep warm.

Apply tourniquet 2-3 inches above wound (or "high and tight" if wound sites undetermined/dynamic scene)

Pack wound cavity tightly with hemostatic impregnated gauze when available, hold direct pressure for 3 minutes

If properly-applied tourniquet is not effective, **apply second tourniquet** side-by-side with the first.

Apply pressure dressing and/or **junctional tourniquet** to maintain hemorrhage control

Continue assessment and care. Treat for shock: lay patient flat, keep warm.

Continue assessment and care. Treat for shock: lay patient flat, keep warm.

Converting "high and tight" tourniquet to 2-3 inches above wound
Expose extremity and identify all wounds. Place second tourniquet 2-3 inches above most proximal wound; tighten and secure. Slowly release proximal tourniquet and assure effectiveness of distal tourniquet. Confirm no bleeding and no distal pulse.

Converting tourniquet to a pressure dressing
Only attempt conversion if: patient is **NOT in shock**, **bleeding has been controlled**, and **time to definitive care is >2 hours.** Conversion must occur within 2 hours of placement of tourniquet and must only be attempted if able to maintain continual monitoring of the extremity. Do not convert tourniquets applied to traumatic amputations. With tourniquet still in place, pack wound and apply pressure dressing. Release tourniquet slowly, assuring that pressure dressing maintains hemorrhage control. Tourniquet must remain in place to be reapplied if rebleeding occurs. If bleeding is not controlled with a pressure dressing (conversion fails) reapply tourniquet.

Transitioning a Tourniquet to a Pressure Dressing

Tourniquet conversion must occur within 2 hours of original placement of the tourniquet and must only be attempted if the ability to maintain continual monitoring of the extremity is possible. Do not convert tourniquets applied to traumatic amputations. Only attempt tourniquet conversion if the patient is **NOT in shock**, bleeding has been controlled, and time to definitive care is anticipated to exceed **2 hours**. While the tourniquet is still in place, pack the wound and apply a pressure dressing. Release the tourniquet and assure that bleeding control is maintained with the pressure dressing. When transitioning to a pressure dressing, the tourniquet should remain around the extremity so as to be easily reapplied if necessary. If bleeding cannot be controlled with a pressure dressing, reapply the tourniquet.

Junctional Bleeding Control

Life-threatening bleeding from areas of the neck, shoulder, armpit, or groin require wound packing due to the inability to apply a tourniquet to these sites. Expose the wound, apply direct pressure, wipe away any pooled blood, and tightly pack gauze (beginning with hemostatic impregnated gauze if available) into the wound while minimizing loss of pressure during your efforts. Focus initial packing efforts on any sites of obvious pulsatile or flowing blood within the wound. Continue to pack the wound cavity tightly with gauze until no further gauze can be pushed into the wound, mound additional gauze over the site, and apply direct pressure using your hands and body weight if required for a minimum of 3 minutes. After 3 minutes apply a modified pressure dressing over the wound if possible and/or a manufactured junctional tourniquet, if available.

Special Considerations

1. Amputations

Definition: A part or all of an extremity that is completely removed from the body.

Treatment: Treat large traumatic amputations by immediately applying a tourniquet 2-3 inches above the amputation site utilizing the previously listed guidelines, and apply an additional pressure dressing to the distal injury. Wrap the amputated appendage in saline-moistened sterile dressings and place in a plastic bag(s). Keep the bag cool but not frozen (ideally in a cooler not in direct contact with ice). Document time of amputation when possible. Initiate rapid evacuation and transport the clearly labeled amputated appendage with the patient.

2. Open Abdominal Injuries

Definition: Evisceration refers to an open abdominal injury in which abdominal contents are exposed and/or protruding from an open wound; this may include the peritoneal lining only or actual organs, such as bowel.

Treatment: Address at "C" after managing massive hemorrhage, airway, and breathing. Position patient supine with knees flexed (if no pelvic or lower extremity fractures). Irrigate grossly-contaminated wounds with clean (potable) water. Moisten large non-stick sterile dressing with sterile water or saline if available; otherwise, moisten with clean (potable) water. Avoid materials that might stick to exposed organs (e.g., paper towels). Carefully apply dressing to exposed organs and cover with occlusive dressing such as Vaseline® gauze, plastic wrap, plastic sandwich bag, or reflective blanket to maintain moisture and warmth. Secure with tape and additional bandaging. Anticipate need to re-moisten dressing during extended care. Treat for shock with special emphasis on maintaining body heat. Avoid giving anything by mouth.

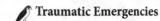

Internal Bleeding

Background

Life-threatening internal bleeding typically occurs in the thoracic, abdominal, and pelvic cavities as a result of direct injury to organs from blunt or penetrating trauma. Each of these cavities can hold multiple liters of blood, and when combined, can easily hold all of the circulating blood volume. Internal bleeding can be **difficult to detect**. Some patients may not exhibit signs and symptoms until a significant amount of internal bleeding has occurred. You must maintain a high index of suspicion for internal bleeding with any patient involved in a significant MOI.

1. **Abdominal Bleeding:** Maintain a high index of suspicion based on MOI.

    Signs and Symptoms: *LOR↓*

    1. Changes in level of responsiveness or altered mental status

    2. Tender, rigid, or distended abdomen

    3. Pain (may be referred to another place in the body. For example, a patient's shoulder may hurt with bleeding around the diaphragm.)

    4. Bruising or discoloration

    5. Signs and symptoms of shock

    6. Bleeding from the urethra, vagina, or rectum

    7. Blood in urine, feces (black, tarry stools), or vomit (coffee-ground appearance)

    Treatment:

    1. ABCDEs.

    2. Avoid giving fluids or food by mouth if not extended patient care.

    3. Consider positioning patient in the recovery position for active or anticipated vomiting, or if a chest injury is suspected.

    4. Position of comfort with preference for keeping the patient flat, typically with knees flexed.

    5. **Keep the patient warm.** Protect the patient from the **environment** by placing them in a hypothermia wrap.

2. **Pelvic Injuries:** A pelvic fracture should be suspected in anyone ejected from a moving vehicle, bucked off a horse, or anyone rolled over by a heavy object like a horse or an ATV. The pelvis typically fractures in numerous places, making the injury physically unstable. Pelvic fractures are extremely painful and may cause significant blood loss. Pelvic injuries should be treated as a circulation problem early in your ABCDE assessment.

    Signs and Symptoms:

    1. Significant pain or tenderness upon palpation to pelvic region

    2. Pelvic instability during physical assessment

    3. Mechanism of injury (MOI) involving blunt force, crushing, ejection, etc.

    4. Signs and symptoms of shock

Treatment:

1. Anticipate and treat for shock

2. Keep the patient warm

3. Minimize rolling the patient or further manipulation of the pelvic region

4. Stabilize the pelvis utilizing a manufactured or improvised pelvic wrap

   - Rotate feet to forward position. Pad space between the legs and buddy splint legs together.

   - Apply pelvic wrap at the level of the greater trochanters (level with the groin).

   - Improvised pelvic wraps can be constructed from backpack hip belts, folded air mattresses (Therm-a-rest™), SAM splints and tourniquet, blankets/sheets, coats or other material, or cut pants. (See page 66)

   - Position and secure the patient to a litter.

   - Provide spinal motion restriction (SMR), when indicated.

Critical Thinking and Evacuation Criteria for Bleeding and Shock

In the civilian (non-combat) world, the vast majority of external bleeds are controllable with a pressure dressing. Massive, life-threatening hemorrhage, such as might be seen from explosions, often require immediate tourniquet application. In a non-military setting, these wounds are relatively rare; in a civilian setting, they may be caused by deep chainsaw injuries, animal attacks, or industrial accidents that cause traumatic amputations.

Because most cases of shock in a civilian setting are due to internal causes such as dehydration and internal bleeding, it is critical to look for and manage early signs and symptoms before your patient decompensates and requires urgent evacuation.

1. Evacuate for all significant bleeds, particularly those that take time to control.
2. Evacuate patients with significant MOI to the abdomen and pelvis.

Evidence base for the recommendations provided in this section and additional resources:

- Wilderness Medical Society Practice Guidelines for Application of Current Hemorrhage Control Techniques for Backcountry Care: Part One, Tourniquets and Hemorrhage Control Adjuncts
- Wilderness Medical Society Practice Guidelines for Application of Current Hemorrhage Control Techniques for Backcountry Care: Part Two, Hemostatic Dressings and Other Adjuncts

Found at: www.aeriemedicine.com/textbook

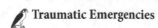
Chest Trauma

Background

WHO: Chest injuries are either a direct cause or a significant factor in 50% of trauma deaths in the United States.

DETAILS: Chest injuries are similarly serious in the backcountry, particularly because the extent of the injury is often initially hidden and the treatment options in the backcountry are extremely limited.

Diagnosis of a specific injury is not usually either important or possible. Instead, it is more important to determine the MOI, to assess the chest for critical injuries, and to recognize signs and symptoms of respiratory distress and internal blood loss. If you are to err, err on the side of assuming the worst and maintain a high index of suspicion during care.

MECHANICS OF BREATHING

During inhalation, the lungs expand and diaphragm contracts, pushing the inferior (bottom) margin of the lungs below the lowest ribs.

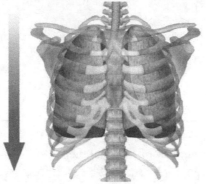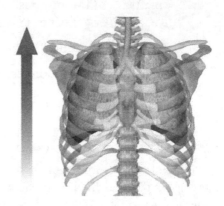

<u>Effective inhalation involves:</u>

1) Diaphragm flattening
2) Ribs rising
3) *Intrathoracic* vacuum

<u>Which requires:</u>

1) Functioning musculature
2) Intact skeleton (ribs)
3) Intact thorax (no holes) maintaining surface tension between the lungs and the thoracic wall lining, the *pleura*

Closed Chest Injuries

1. Isolated Rib Fractures or Bruises

Injuries resulting in pain <u>without</u> <u>obvious</u> ABCDE problems

1. **Definition:** Fractured or bruised ribs without an open chest wound or flail segment (see flail chest for more details).

2. **Signs and Symptoms:** Pain with inspiration, coughing, laughing or other movement; crepitus, point tenderness, self-splinting with arm on affected side.

3. **Treatment:**
   - ABCDEs
   - Position of comfort
   - Splint the arm on the injured side (taping over the ribs rarely helps and may lead to pneumonia)

2. Multiple Rib Fractures or Flail Chest

Injuries Resulting in Pain <u>with</u> ABCDE Problems

1. **Definition:** Two or more adjacent ribs broken in two or more places. **This is MUCH more dangerous than an isolated rib fracture.**

2. **Signs and Symptoms:** Difficulty breathing, paradoxical chest wall movement, often accompanied by shock and severe respiratory distress.

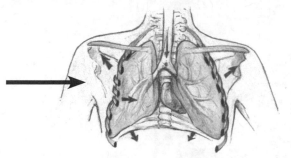

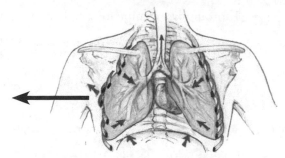

Paradoxical movement of flail chest during <u>inspiration</u>

Paradoxical movement of flail chest during <u>exhalation</u>

3. **Treatment:**
- ABCDEs
- Stabilize the flail segment with bulky padded dressing
- Position the patient on the injured side if the patient can tolerate it, or place in a position of comfort

3. Simple Pneumothorax
Closed Injuries Resulting in Difficulty Breathing

1. **Definition**: Air in a closed chest cavity may cause the lung on the affected side to collapse due to the loss of vacuum attaching it to chest wall. This can occur with or without trauma.

2. **Signs and Symptoms:** Shortness of breath, rapid heart rate, pain

3. **Treatment:**
- ABCDEs
- Position of comfort
- Keep injured side down

4. Closed Hemothorax
Closed Injuries Resulting in Shock

1. **Definition:** Blood collecting in the chest cavity.

2. **Signs and Symptoms:** Shortness of breath, rapid heart rate, shock, production of bloody or pink tinged sputum.

3. **Treatment:**
- ABCDEs
- Treat for Shock

Open Chest Injuries

5. Sucking Chest Wound
Open Chest Wound with Difficulty Breathing

1. **Definition:** Air in an open chest cavity leads to the lung on the affected side to collapse due to the displacement of the vacuum with air from the outside entering through an open chest wound.

2. **Signs and Symptoms:** Shortness of breath, rapid heart rate, rapid/shallow respirations, possible air exchange at the injury site (known as a "sucking chest wound").

3. **Treatment:**
- ABCDEs
- Initially the open chest wound should be covered with a gloved hand followed by a 3-sided occlusive dressing or manufactured vented chest seal.

- Thoroughly examine for a potential exit wound.

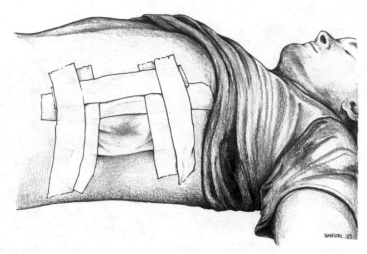

Three-sided occlusive dressing for "sucking chest wounds"

6. Tension Pneumothorax

1. **Definition:** Air is trapped within the thoracic cavity with increasing pressure, eventually putting pressure on the other thoracic organs (in particular, the heart and great vessels). Unmitigated, it will lead to shock and kill the patient.

2. **Signs and Symptoms:** Difficulty breathing, tracheal deviation (a very late sign), S/S of shock

3. **Treatment:**
   - ABCDEs.
   - If the patient has a "sucking chest wound," secure a 3-sided occlusive dressing or manufactured chest seal for efficacy; "burp" the dressing if necessary.

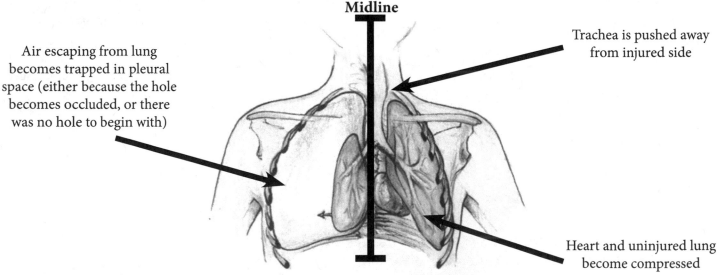

Midline

Air escaping from lung becomes trapped in pleural space (either because the hole becomes occluded, or there was no hole to begin with)

Trachea is pushed away from injured side

Heart and uninjured lung become compressed

7. Impaled Object in the Chest Wall

1. **Definition:** Any object that enters the chest cavity.

2. **Signs and Symptoms:** Shortness of breath, pain, possible sucking chest wound, tension pneumothorax.

3. **Treatment:**
   - ABCDEs.
   - Stabilize the object in place.
   - Carefully shorten the object if it cannot be splinted or it prevents a safe evacuation.
   - Treat for sucking chest wound.

Critical Thinking and Evacuation Criteria for Chest Trauma

Most of the important structures in the chest are hidden from view and therefore difficult to assess. Keep things simple: If there is a hole in the chest wall, cover it with a three-sided dressing or manufactured vented chest seal; if the chest wall shows signs of trauma, put the patient in the position that makes breathing easiest, and if they don't have a preference, try to keep the injured side down by positioning the patient on their injured side. On the more subtle side, look for signs and symptoms of blood loss and difficulty breathing. If you see any of these, evacuate. Specifically:

1. **Rapidly evacuate** patients with signs/symptoms of:

   - Multiple rib fractures or flail chest

   - Hemothorax

   - Pneumothorax

   - Open chest injuries ("sucking chest wound")

   - Tension pneumothorax

   - Impalements to the chest wall

2. **Evacuate** patients with significant chest-wall trauma - fractures, large bruises, penetrating wounds and/or intolerable pain.

3. **Evacuate** patients with MOI and signs and symptoms of respiratory distress, including an inability to breathe deeply or comfortably.

4. **Evacuate** patients with MOI and signs and symptoms of blood loss.

5. **Evacuate** patients whose compromised respiratory status will decrease their ability to move to the point that group safety is jeopardized.

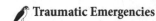

Head Injuries

Background

WHO: Roughly 50% of trauma deaths in the U.S. are due to head injuries. They are the leading cause of death in persons 1-42 years old.

DETAILS: Head injuries are difficult to assess and manage in the backcountry. Severe head injuries require intensive medical care at an appropriate facility.

PREVENTION: Wear a helmet and seat belts. Remain within your skill level in any activity.

Signs and Symptoms of Head Injuries

1. Altered Level of Responsiveness (LOR) is the hallmark of brain injury (<u>D</u>isoriented, <u>I</u>rritable, <u>C</u>ombative)
2. Repetitive questioning and/or inability to recall recent events
3. Nausea, vomiting
4. Fatigue
5. Headache
6. Blood or cerebrospinal fluid (CSF) from ears or nose
7. Seizures
-------------- Signs of increasing intracranial pressure (ICP) --------------
8. Battle's sign or raccoon eyes
9. Unequal pupils
10. Posturing (involuntary flexion or extension of muscles)
11. Decreasing heart rate (a late, less reliable sign that may be preceded by increasing heart rates)
12. Increasing blood pressure (without a BP cuff this may be identified by increasingly strong peripheral pulses)
13. Changes in respiratory pattern – Rapid or irregular breathing

Treatment for Head Injuries

1. ABCDEs. Establish, maintain, and diligently reassess. Anticipate vomiting, seizures, and changes in LOR.
2. Provide spinal motion restriction (SMR). Determine the need to maintain SMR utilizing SMR criteria.

Mild injuries (mild symptoms that decrease over time)

1. Monitor hourly for 24 hours for signs of worsening signs and symptoms.
2. Evacuate, particularly if the patient is your client or vital signs deteriorate (especially LOR).

Severe Injuries (increasing symptoms)

1. Provide spinal motion restriction. Maintain the head in an in-line, neutral position.
2. Head injuries require aggressive airway management; diligently establish and maintain an open airway.
3. Assist ventilations if respirations are inadequate. *Episodes of decreased oxygenation increase mortality.*
4. Monitor vital signs and patient condition carefully.
   - If S/S of shock/low BP (weak, rapid pulses): maintain spinal motion restriction. Position with the head level with the body, supine or in the recovery position. *Episodes of low BP increase mortality.*
   - If S/S of increasing ICP: While maintaining spinal motion restriction, elevate the head and torso on an incline or by flexing at the waist to 15-30 degrees. Maintain neutral in-line positioning of the head, un-shrug shoulders, eliminate constriction around the neck, and protect from lights and noise.

Critical Thinking and Evacuation Criteria for Head Injuries

It can be difficult to identify the severity of a head injury based on a patient's initial presentation. While they can be delayed longer, S/S usually manifest within the first 24 hours after injury. Don't wait until you have an altered or unresponsive, seizing, vomiting patient to initiate evacuation and seek further help.

1. **Evacuate** any head trauma patient that results in loss or change of responsiveness.
2. **Evacuate** any head trauma patient on blood thinners (Coumadin/Warfarin, etc.).

Spinal Injuries

Background

WHO: The World Health Organization reports 250,000 to 500,000 annual incidents of new spinal cord injuries internationally. The National Spinal Cord Injury Statistical Center reports approximately 17,000 new spinal cord injuries in the U.S. each year. Young adults and the elderly make up the majority of incidents; the elderly may experience injury more easily than younger counterparts. Vehicle crashes are the leading cause of injury followed by falls, acts of violence, and sports/recreational activities. Sporting injuries globally account for between 7% and 18% of all spinal cord injuries.

PREVENTION: Always wear a seat belt (including when traveling abroad) and other PPE when appropriate, observe the speed limit, utilize extra caution when driving in inclement weather and terrain, and maintain zero tolerance for drinking and driving. Practice good risk management and maintain an awareness of party member's skill level when participating in activities with the potential for falls or high speed impact such as climbing, biking, horseback riding, winter sports, water sports, and off road travel.

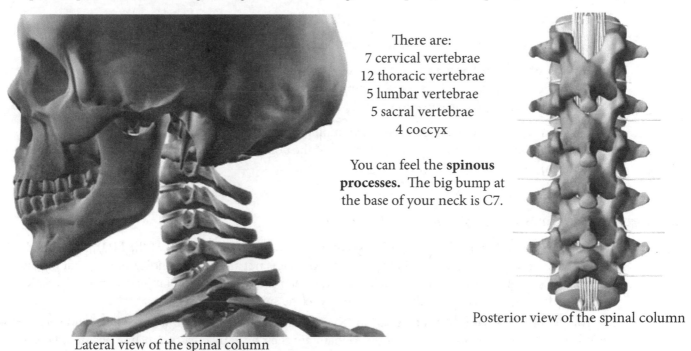

There are:
7 cervical vertebrae
12 thoracic vertebrae
5 lumbar vertebrae
5 sacral vertebrae
4 coccyx

You can feel the **spinous processes.** The big bump at the base of your neck is C7.

Posterior view of the spinal column

Lateral view of the spinal column

ANATOMY AND PHYSIOLOGY: The **spinal column** is made up of 26 vertebrae that extend from the base of the skull to the pelvis. There are 7 cervical vertebrae (C1-C7), 12 thoracic (T1-T12), and 5 lumbar (L1-L5); 5 fused vertebrae make up the sacrum, which forms the posterior portion of the pelvis. An additional 4 fused vertebrae form the coccyx, the lower end of the spine.

Enclosed in the spinal column is the **spinal cord**, a delicate organ composed of nervous tissue that extends from the brain stem to approximately L2. With the brain, it makes up the **central nervous system** (CNS).

The **peripheral nervous system** (PNS) is made up of nerves found outside the spinal column which communicate impulses to and from the CNS. We assess **motor, pain, and light touch tracts** of the nervous system by performing a CSM check on all extremities.

Spinal column injury typically results in pain or tenderness to the spine. **Spinal cord injury** can result in abnormal motor and/or sensory function. Spinal column injury can occur without spinal cord injury and conversely, spinal cord injury may occur without spinal column injury. Either will be referred to as a **spinal injury**. Signs and symptoms of potential spinal column injury are much more common than actual spinal cord injury.

Sign and Symptoms of Spinal Injuries

1. Midline neck or back pain.

2. Midline neck or back tenderness (pain upon palpation).

3. Abnormal sensation in one or more extremities (numbness, tingling, weakness, abnormal CSM and/or inability to feel light touch, sharp touch, and/or pain).

4. Abnormality or inequality in extremity motor function (grip strength, foot strength).

-------------- Less common, but more definitive findings --------------------

5. Complete or partial paralysis of the upper and/or lower extremities.

6. Bruising and/or crepitus.

7. Deformity to the spine (step-off deformity, swelling, indention)

8. Loss of bladder and/or bowel control (due to loss of motor control).

9. Priapism (sustained erection of the penis due to dilation of vessels below spinal cord injury).

10. Abnormal respiratory effort due to disruption of nerve impulses to the muscles of breathing.

11. Low blood pressure noted as weak or absent distal pulses. This is due to vasodilation from disruption of nerve impulses which maintain vasomotor tone; typically accompanied by flushed skin below the injury and low to normal heart rate.

12. Signs and Symptoms of a significant head injury (although significant head injuries can occur without injury to the spine, we cannot rule out the potential for a spinal injury in the unreliable head-injured patient).

Treatment for Spinal Injuries

1. Maintain a high index of suspicion for spinal injuries based on evaluation of the **MOI**. Although MOI should lead you to initiate spinal motion restriction, it is not an accurate indicator of spinal injury. A fall from standing with a well-placed blow to the head can result in spinal injury; conversely, patients can fall from great height resulting in no injury to the spine.

2. Provide initial **spinal motion restriction** (SMR) with manual stabilization of the head and neck ("Hold C-Spine") and/or encourage the patient to maintain their head in a neutral in-line position. Due to the pain of a spinal injury, a reliable patient typically will not move their head to the point of causing further harm. The goal of SMR is to *minimize unwanted movement of the potentially injured spine.*

3. Perform a **Primary Survey** and correct **ABCDEs** problems. Do not allow prioritization of manual stabilization to distract you from performing the more important task of assessing for and correcting life-threatening scene safety or ABCDE problems.

4. If you have initiated SMR, evaluate further need to do so by completing a secondary survey and utilize the **SMR criteria**. Indications for continued SMR following blunt trauma include any of the following:

   a. **Unreliable patient**: Altered level of responsiveness or a loss of consciousness from the event (not alert and oriented x 4, evidence of intoxication); distracting injuries or circumstances (long bone fracture, degloving, crush injuries, large burns, emotional distress, communication barrier)

   b. **Midline spinal pain and/or tenderness**

   c. **Deformity of the spine**

   d. **Neurologic deficits** (numbness, weakness, abnormal sensations)

   If the patient is 100% reliable and has no signs and symptoms of spinal injury, SMR is not indicated.

5. Realign the head and neck to a **neutral, in-line position:**

   a. A neutral, in-line position is the preferred position for a patient with suspected spinal injury. This means the head is facing forward with the nose in-line with the umbilicus and is neither flexed forward nor extended backwards. This allows for better airway management, increased comfort, and may help avoid worsening symptoms.

   b. Perform realignment carefully, one axis at a time. Stop if the patient experiences an increase in pain or resistance is felt.

   c. Positioning may initially be maintained by **manual stabilization**. Consider application of a manufactured or improvised cervical collar such as the "Montana horse collar" while maintaining manual stabilization. Carefully place padding under and around the head to maintain positioning.

      Use of rigid cervical collars is controversial but remains a standard of care as one component of SMR in many EMS systems. The use of a rigid collar device must be undertaken with caution and strict avoidance of harm (airway compromise, aspiration, pain, pressure sores, increased intracranial pressure, and increased movement or extension of the head and neck).

   d. If pain or resistance prevents realignment, maintain manual stabilization while improvising materials to assist in maintaining the position; it may be incredibly challenging to maintain SMR in this scenario.

6. The remainder of the spine should be stabilized keeping the **head, neck, and torso aligned**. The method utilized should be comfortable and conform to the patient (the patient should not be made to conform to a device). This can be accomplished by positioning the patient on their back, on their back with head and torso elevated 15-45 degrees, or on their side. When available utilize a manufactured vacuum mattress designed for SMR.

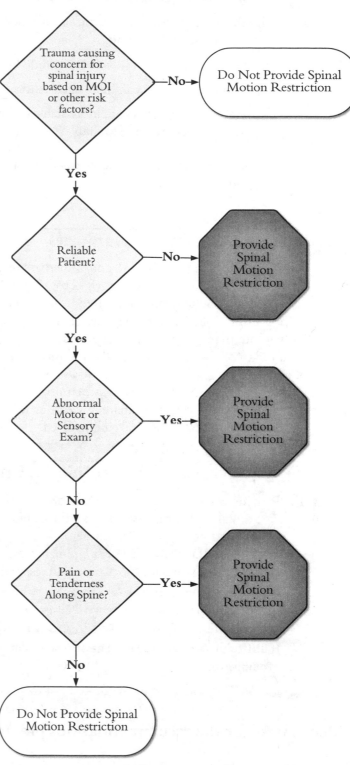

Unless specified by local or institutional protocols, we do not recommend the use of a traditional backboard other than as an extrication device or to assist in moving patients short distances. Except in circumstances where in-line positioning of the head cannot otherwise be maintained, we do not recommend the routine taping of the patient's head to a device.

7. **Special attention** should be taken to maintain the head, neck, and torso in alignment during any patient moves. Adequate padding must be provided for immobile patients. Movement of the patient with potential spinal injury can be accomplished as follows:

   a. A reliable patient, who is able to do so, may self-extricate from a vehicle, or small or otherwise unsafe space after placement of a collar device.

   b. Short moves from one surface to another should ideally be performed utilizing a lift and slide technique or BEAMing.

   c. Log rolling can be utilized, but should be limited in frequency with suspected spinal injuries.

   d. Improvised litters can be invaluable for moving patients, preferably for shorter distances.

   e. Manufactured litters are more stable and often designed for specific rescue environment, generally making them the most reliable.

8. SMR is not indicated for patients who have suffered isolated penetrating trauma to the neck or torso (i.e., gunshot wounds, stabbings).

Critical Thinking for Spinal Injuries

Much has changed in both EMS and wilderness medicine regarding best practices for suspected spinal injury. While it is clear that rigid backboards and collars do little to protect spines and often cause harm (including but not limited to airway compromise, aspiration, respiratory compromise, pain, pressure sores, increased intracranial pressure, and worsening alignment of the spine), we are left without many alternatives that are based on good evidence. In no other instance will rescuers be required to consider more carefully the risks and benefits of their actions. A wilderness evacuation of a patient with spinal motion restriction poses substantial risks to patients and rescuers. Walking a patient with an unstable cervical fracture out of the backcountry is also risky. The gravity of the decisions required can overwhelm any care provider. Use your best judgment to determine an evacuation plan that is safest for all involved.

Evacuation Criteria for Spinal Injuries Utilizing Spinal Motion Restriction (SMR):

1. Patients who meet criteria for maintaining SMR should be **evacuated** to definitive care. Deciding by what means (assisting the ambulatory patient vs. litter carry) requires a detailed understanding of the MOI, a systematic assessment of both the patient and environment, and must weigh the goals of SMR *(minimizing unwanted movement of the potentially injured spine)* against the risk to both the patient and rescuers.

2. Consider allowing the reliable ambulatory patient with no neurologic deficits to self-extricate and potentially **self-evacuate with assistance**. This does not come without risk to the patient, so this option must be weighed against the risk of additional injury to the patient and/or rescuers.

3. If SMR does not put the patient or rescuers at greater risk, the prudent choice is **litter evacuation**.

Evidence base for the recommendations provided in this section and additional resources:

- Wilderness Medical Society Practice Guidelines for Spine Immobilization in the Austere Environment: 2014 Update

Found at: www.aeriemedicine.com/textbook

Open Wounds

Background

For the purpose of brevity, the following discussions about wound management assume that the wound is isolated and is not causing life-threatening bleeding. This is not a reasonable assumption to make in the field: it must be proven with a thorough and systematic physical assessment.

DEFINITION: An **open wound** is a break in the skin, ranging from a superficial abrasion to a deep laceration.

Important Medical History

- Determine whether the patient is taking blood thinners, as these will significantly delay blood clotting.
- Determine whether the patient has diabetes or recent immunosuppressive therapy such as cancer treatment that will delay healing and make them more prone to infections.
- Confirm that the patient has been immunized for tetanus.
- Note rabies vaccination status for any animal bites.

Treatment

Immediate Priorities

1. Control significant bleeding.
2. Protect yourself with gloves, glasses, clothing, etc.
3. Identify high-risk wounds.
4. Reduce discomfort and maintain function.

Long-term Care

Clean the wound

1. Reduce the risk of infection and promote tissue healing

2. Prepare your area and necessary supplies: BSI, water in a single-use container, instruments, dressings, etc. Avoid splashback and saturating your patient. Wound care requires "clean" technique, sterility is not necessary.

3. If the wound is bleeding lightly, don't be overly concerned about stopping the bleed. Instead, inspect the wound for debris, impaled objects, and damaged anatomy.

> **High-Risk Wounds**
>
> › **Bites**
> › **Grossly contaminated/ dirty wounds**
> › **Exposed bone, ligament, tendon, joint capsule, fat or muscle**
> › **Deep punctures**
> › **Crushing injuries**
> › **Gaping wounds**
> › **Wounds to high-risk patients (e.g., diabetics, immunosuppressive medications/therapies)**

4. Use clean (potable/drinkable) water to clean in and around the wound.

   - **Do not** use additives such as povidone-iodine, chlorhexidine gluconate, benzalkonium chloride, hydrogen peroxide, or soap for wound irrigation (except in the case of possible rabies exposure). While effective in decreasing initial bacterial counts in wounds, these agents are also toxic to tissue, causing increased healing complications and rebound bacterial counts after 48 hours.

   - As an exception, wounds with a high risk of rabies exposure should be cleaned with soap and water and irrigated with a virucidal agent such as povidone-iodine or chlorine dioxide.

4. Use high volume (1 liter or more), high pressure (6-12 psi) irrigation to help remove foreign matter and reduce the bacteria count within the wound. This is best accomplished using an irrigation syringe. *Although irrigation should not take priority over assessment and care of immediate concerns, it should be performed as quickly as practical to maximize effectiveness.*

5. Use tweezers or sterile gauze to pick out embedded particles. Use your judgment with the amount of pressure/scrubbing needed, taking care not to push debris further into the wound.

6. Visually inspect the wound closely for remaining foreign particles. The wound should be as free as possible of debris.
   - You may cause further bleeding by poking through loose tissue, irrigating under flaps of skin (avulsions), or scrubbing with gauze. If the initial bleeding was minor, it should be relatively minor capillary bleeding. However, if bleeding is significant, control with direct pressure.

Consider closing LOW-RISK wounds

No decision to attempt wound closure should be made in haste and no closed wound should be left unattended.

1. After the bleeding is controlled and the wound is thoroughly cleaned and irrigated, clip hair from inside and around the wound if necessary.
   - Do not shave hair at wound edges, as this irritates and abrades the skin and causes infection.

2. Tissue adhesives may be considered to close minor, low-tension wounds.

3. Apply tincture of benzoin (after asking if the patient has allergies) to either side of the wound. Do not place benzoin in a wound.

4. Approximate the wound edges, making them touch each other, with Steri-strips™, butterfly bandages, or an improvised closure strip. Avoid misalignment and bunching of wound edges by beginning in the middle of the wound and working outward to either end. Do not cause shear stress or stretching of the skin.

5. Consider antibiotic cream or ointment over wound.

6. Dress the wound (see below).

7. If signs of infection develop, consider removing attempts at wound closure to allow reopening of the wound and treat for infection (see below).

NOTE: Consider closing only if the wound is small, clean, and otherwise not at high risk for infection. Wound edges should be smooth and not jagged or irregular.

Leave open HIGH-RISK wounds

1. Clean as previously described.

2. If large, pack with moist (not dripping) sterile gauze.

3. Dress wound (see below). Pack wounds with exposed tissues or bone with moist dressings.

4. Change packing daily and consider Steri-strips™ to approximate wound edges after five days without infection.

5. Consider antibiotics.

6. Evacuate patient.

NOTE: Remember, scar revisions can successfully disguise scars weeks after the injury. So, be conservative when deciding whether or not to close a wound.

Dress the Wound

1. Apply a slightly moist, sterile dressing which helps promote wound healing and a clean bandage to secure and further protect the dressing site (not as tight as a pressure dressing).
   - Dressings are the initial covering on a wound such as a sterile gauze pad, 4x4, or Tegaderm™, a semi-permeable membrane.
   - Consider covering with non-stick dressing such as Spyroflex™ or Telfa™. (For abrasions, Second Skin™ or Telfa™ work well.)
   - Bandages by definition are not in direct contact with the wound, but instead hold dressings in place.

Signs and Symptoms of Infection

LOCALIZED

- Redness surrounding the wound
- Pus in wound

TRANSITION

- Heat at wound site
- Swelling beyond wound site
- Lymphatic streaking
- Lymphatic swelling proximal to wound
- Increasing local heat
- Increasing pain beyond wound

lymphatic ~ towards

SYSTEMIC

- Weakness
- Chills, fever
- Nausea, vomiting

Signs of Sepsis (in the presence of a known or suspected source of infection)

- Decreased/altered LOR
- Elevated RR (> 22 bpm)
- Elevated HR (> 90 bpm)
- Decreased BP (< 100 mmHg)
- Temperature higher than 100.4°F (38°C) or lower than 96.8°F (36°C)

Treatment for Infected Small Wounds

1. Clean the wound (this may require removing the scab).
2. Heat compresses and/or hot water soaks 3 times per day for 20 minutes.
3. Splint and immobilize if on an extremity.
4. Consider antibiotics.

Evacuation Criteria for Open Wounds

1. **Rapidly evacuate** if wounds are associated with signs of systemic infection (fever, chills, weakness).
2. **Rapidly evacuate** for signs of sepsis in the presence of known or suspected source of infection.
3. **Evacaute** if wounds will not heal despite continued appropriate care.

○ Only pop friction blisters

Specific Wounds

1. Hot Spots and Blisters

blister is about to form

Definition: A **hot spot** is the warm painful telltale sign of an impending blister. A **blister** is fluid that has collected within the layers of skin as a result of *moisture*, *heat*, and *friction*.

Prevention: Stay hydrated, maintain adequate nutrition and form. Keep your toenails trimmed and calluses filed. Keep your feet **dry** and **reduce friction** with a personalized combination of the following: proper fitting and broken-in footwear (laced correctly), single or double-layered synthetic or wool blended moisture-wicking socks (avoid cotton), well conditioned feet, gaiters, anti-perspirants, foot lubricants or powders, skin-toughening products, and the appropriate use of blister dressings, MoleSkin™, Leukotape™, and/or duct tape.

Signs and Symptoms

1. Patient feels a hot spot or sharp burning sensation as the blister is formed.
2. Bubble of skin containing fluid that might be accompanied by pain, redness, or itching.

Treatment

1. Protect hot spots and provide pressure relief with tape, blister dressings, or donut-shaped pads. Smaller blisters (<5 mm) can be protected similarly to hot spots.
2. Drain larger blisters (>5 mm) while leaving the skin in place. Avoid draining blisters in diabetics and other high risk patients.
3. Clean the blister and the area around it well.
4. Use a sterile needle to pierce the lower edge of the blister.
5. Apply pressure to disperse the fluid, while attempting to not allow air to enter the space.
6. Once the fluid is removed, clean the area and consider covering with an antibiotic ointment.
7. Cover the blister with a friction-resistant dressing to prevent infection and further damage. Moleskin™ donuts, Second Skin™, Tegaderm™, Leukotape™, and duct tape all work well. If skin is accidentally removed, treat as an abrasion or open wound. Place a doughnut pad around the dressed blister to avoid further irritation.
8. Tips before applying tape or other dressings to your feet: wipe the area with an alcohol pad to clean and remove oils, apply tincture of benzoin to assist adhesion, and round the corners of your tape by trimming with scissors; tape corners have a tendency to catch and peel inside your sock.

2. Contusions

Definition: Bruising with no break in the skin. Mechanisms of injury include a direct or crushing force.

Signs and Symptoms

1. The pain from a contusion may mimic a fracture. If in doubt, treat the injury as a fracture.
2. These types of injuries **swell**, sometimes far more than what you might expect. Bruising a bone near a joint may cause significant inflammation of the joint.

Treatment

1. **First 48 Hours:** Rest, ice (20-30 minutes every 2 hours), compression, elevation. Ice should not be directly applied to the skin.
2. **After 48-72 Hours:** Warm packs 2-3 times daily for 15-20 minutes, compression, pain-free activity.
3. Consider ibuprofen or other non-steroidal anti-inflammatory drugs (NSAIDs). Be sure to ask if there are allergies to recommended medication.

3. Eviscerated Organs

Definition: Abdominal contents are exposed and protruding from an open wound.

Signs and Symptoms

1. Visualization of abdominal organs through an open wound.

Treatment

1. Moisten sterile dressing. If available, use sterile water.
2. Apply dressing to wound and cover with occlusive dressing such as Vaseline® gauze or plastic wrap to keep organs from drying out. (See page 37)

4. Impaled Objects

Definition: Object that punctures the skin or tissue and is left in place.

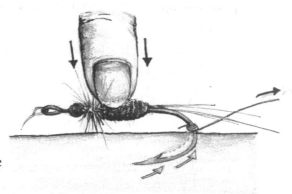

Signs and Symptoms

- Visualization of object protruding from a wound.

Treatment

- Most impaled objects should be left in place. Notable exceptions include objects that occlude (block) the airway, those that interfere with the function and therefore a risk to life, and those that can be easily removed (e.g., fish hooks).
- Stabilize object.
- If possible, cut the object to avoid unnecessary movement.

Fishhook Removal:
Add light pressure down and tug, or jerk, the line *quickly* to get most hooks out.
DO NOT TRY THIS ON AN EYE, and protect your own while doing it.

Critical Thinking for Managing Open Wounds

Most open wounds are easily managed and do not require evacuation. While minor wounds can be managed in the backcountry, they are often overlooked and can become life threats. Pay attention to all wounds and be vigilant with their care.

Critical Thinking and Evacuation Criteria for All Wounds

At some level, all wounds are colonized by outside organisms and are therefore "infected". The body handles most wounds without assistance. In a remote setting, however, our hygiene is often questionable and our margin of error is slim, so assistance should always be given by minimizing contamination and monitoring for an infection that could make your patient sick.

1. **Evacuate** if wound shows any signs or symptoms beyond localized infection.
2. **Evacuate** if wound shows no signs of improvement over time.
3. **Evacuate** for contusions with suspected underlying fractures or contusions with significant MOI.
4. **Evacuate** any impaled object or evisceration.
5. **Evacuate** if the patient shows any signs or symptoms of shock due to internal/external bleeding or sepsis.

Head, Eyes, Ears, Nose and Throat (HEENT)

DETAILS: Injuries to the scalp, face, eyes, ears, nose and teeth are common and painful. Because these areas are heavily vascularized and innervated, they may bleed profusely and hurt a lot.

In general, treatment for these wounds includes stopping the bleeding and preventing infection. However, always check for underlying fractures and maintain an index of suspicion for c-spine injury.

1. Scalp Injuries

Special Concerns: Lacerations to the scalp bleed a lot. The primary concerns are underlying brain injury, blood loss, and shock, but a related secondary concern is getting wet and potentially hypothermic.

Treatment

- Stop the bleeding with direct pressure.
- Consider MOI and suspect spinal and head injuries.

2. Nose Bleeds

Causes: Environmental (altitude and dry air), medications (blood thinners/aspirin), disease (high blood pressure or clotting disorders) or trauma.

Special Concerns: Be suspicious of head injury with bleeding from the nose in a trauma patient, especially if the MOI suggests a direct force to the nose/face.

Prevention: Hydration, the use of Vaseline® to lubricate the inner part of the nostril, or breathing through a handkerchief in dry environments are ways to prevent nose bleeds.

Treatment

- Consider the MOI and suspect spinal and head injuries.
- If non-trauma/spontaneous nose bleed, have the patient sit up and lean slightly forward. Then pinch the soft part of the nose just below the bone for at least 10 minutes. Do not attempt if nasal bone fractures are suspected.
- A rolled tissue plug partially inserted into the nostril helps control blood flow after the bleeding has mostly stopped. Removing may cause further bleeding.
- Monitor for airway compromise.

3. Teeth Injuries

Special Concerns: Assess and monitor the patient's airway! Significant tooth pain is often unbearable. Teeth may be cracked or knocked out. This can be extremely painful.

Prevention: Take care of your teeth. Visit the dentist before leaving on extended trips.

Treatment

- Consider the MOI and suspect spinal and head injuries.
- For simple pain and sensitivity without trauma (e.g., general toothache), consider soaking gauze with clove oil (eugenol) and placing around/in an affected tooth.
- If tooth is completely avulsed (partially or completely knocked out), clean tooth and socket *gently*, particularly to remove blood clots from the socket. Replace tooth into socket. The tooth has a good chance of being re-implanted if the patient visits an oral surgeon within 30 minutes. Buddy-splint unstable teeth in place with dental floss or softened candle-wax.
- If tooth is not replaceable into socket and patient is fully conscious, place in gauze/ cotton and put back in patient's mouth (like chewing tobacco).

- If this is not possible or the tooth is partially avulsed, cover socket or exposed area with dental filling paste, moist gauze, Cavit® Temporary Filling Material, or wax (melted but cool candle wax will work).

- Minor bleeding can be controlled with direct pressure or the application of a moist black or green tea bag. Leave it on for 20-30 minutes.

- Watch for signs and symptoms of infection, such as pain when speaking, opening the mouth, or swallowing, and fever.

4. Eye Injuries

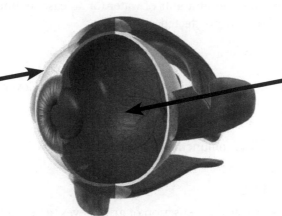

The cornea, or white of an eye, is easily scratched and even sunburned (snowblindness). *It is incredibly sensitive.* Contact lens wearers are at increased risk for problems.

The inside of an eyeball is filled with fluid (the humors), that keeps the ball round and allow us to see.

1. Foreign Bodies
Treatment
- Do not rub the eye.
- Gently irrigate the eye with large quantities of clean water or saline solution. Irrigate away from the healthy, uninjured eye.
- If the above doesn't work, roll the eyelid back using a cotton swab and remove the object with clean, moistened gauze.
- If you are unable to remove it, cover **both** eyes and evacuate.
- Do not attempt removal of impaled objects.

2. Impaled Object
Treatment
- Stabilize in place with moist, sterile cloth and cover both eyes to prevent eyeball movement.

3. Corneal Abrasions
Signs and Symptoms: Pain similar to that of snow blindness, the feeling of something burning or abrading the eye. Sometimes it itches and blinking may hurt.

Treatment
- Apply cool compresses.
- Evaluate for foreign bodies and assess for infection (green pus, increasing pain, change in vision, redness).
- Sterile saline eye drops may provide comfort.
- Consider topical ophthalmic antibiotics, such as tobramycin ophthalmic solution for infection.
- If available, consider topical tetracaine to numb the eye. This is safe to use every 30 minutes while awake, for up to 24 hours.

4. Avulsed Eyeball

Treatment

- **Do not** return the eyeball to the socket.
- Wrap the eye with dressing moistened with sterile saline solution and protect the injury. If the evacuation is long, continue to keep the dressing moist.

5. Burns to the Eye

Chemical Burns

Treatment: Flush with copious amounts of water for at least 20 minutes. Hold the eyelid open and flush away from the unaffected eye.

Thermal Burns

Treatment: Stop the burning process by flushing with water. Cover the eye with saline-moistened sterile dressing.

Snowblindness - UV burn of the conjunctivae (mucus membrane of the eye).

Signs and Symptoms

- Sensitivity to light.
- Pain with eye movement, sensation of grit in eyes (assess for foreign objects in the eye).
- Reddened conjunctivae.

Treatment

- Apply cool moist cloth to eyelids. Consider sterile saline eye drops for comfort.
- Place patient in dark space. Keep eyes protected from further UV exposure.
- Consider pain medications such as ibuprofen, as necessary.

Evacuation Criteria for HEENT Injuries

1. **Rapid evacuation** for impaled objects, avulsed eyeballs, or misshaped or leaking eyeballs.
2. **Evacuate** patients with foreign bodies in the eyes that cannot be easily removed.
3. **Evacuate** chemical and thermal burns to eyes.
4. **Evacuate** gross or persistent visual changes.
5. **Evacuate** eye injuries with pain or irritation worsening over 24 hours.
6. **Evacuate** scalp, nose, dental, or eye injuries with significant bleeding, particularly those that take time to control.
7. **Evacuate** any scalp, nose, dental, or eye injuries associated with significant MOI or suspected spinal or head injury.
8. **Evacuate** if the patient shows signs or symptoms of shock due to blood loss.
9. **Evacuate** if the patient shows signs and symptoms of infection or sepsis.
10. **Evacuate** for avulsed or partially avulsed teeth.
11. **Evacuate** any HEENT injury associated with altered LOC or ability to control their own airway.

Burns

Background

PREVALENCE: Large, life-threatening burns are relatively uncommon in the backcountry. The most common types of burns in the backcountry are small, isolated thermal burns or sunburns, requiring long-term care rather than evacuation. Chemical burns or larger thermal burns require evacuation to definitive care.

PHYSIOLOGY: Burns destroy tissue and cause inflammation, fluid loss, and loss of thermal control. Because burns destroy the body's protective barrier, they are easily infected and are a prime source for systemic infection.

PREVENTION: One of the most common causes of burns in the backcountry is a camp stove accident. Always put stoves on as flat and secure a surface as possible and wear only closed-toed shoes around a stove. Use sunscreen and/or protective UV clothing to prevent sunburn.

Signs/Symptoms and Assessment of Burns

Location: Part of body on which the burn occurred – identify high-risk areas (e.g., face, hands, etc.).

Extent: Estimate extent of burn – patient's palm is approximately 1% of their body surface area (BSA).

Depth

1. **Superficial**:

   - Local pain and tenderness, redness (e.g., sunburn).
   - No blebs or blisters.

2. **Partial-Thickness**:

   - Blister formation is key criteria.
   - Shallow: wet, red, painful blisters.
   - Deep: dry, mottled, partially painful blisters.

3. **Full-Thickness**:

   - The skin is charred through to the tissues that underlie it.
   - Skin may appear red, black, or white and waxy. Wound is dry and hard.
   - No pain at the wound site, but very painful surrounding it. "Bulls-eye" pattern of depth: full-thickness in center, partial thickness surrounding that, to superficial around the edges.

Treatment (Specific Burns)

Thermal Burns

1. **Stop the burning process.**
   - Safely remove smoldering clothing and jewelry. These items may cause circulation constriction as swelling occurs.
   - Douse with water. Be wary of inducing hypothermia in your patient. For pain control this may be continued for upwards of ½ hour.
2. Gently cleanse with potable water.
3. Apply aloe (with no additives) for superficial burns.
4. Cover with **slightly moist**, sterile dressings.
   - Separate digits of hands or feet when dressing.
   - Wrap bandages loosely and keep slightly moist.
6. Do not pop closed blisters.
7. If the burn is small, cover with non-adhesive dressing.

8. Elevate and consider ibuprofen to reduce swelling.

9. Have patient gently and regularly move burned area.

10. As their airway permits, maintain patient hydration, so that they are urinating clearly and copiously.

11. If evacuation will occur within 24 hours, do not redress wound. Otherwise, if supplies are available, change dressings every other day (soak off old dressings with cool, clean water).

Sunburns

Prevention is most important

- Reduce ultraviolet (UV) exposure between 9 am and 3 pm.

- Increase awareness and avoidance at elevation.

- Increase awareness with sensitive skin types (those on certain medications, particularly some antibiotics, and younger individuals).

Treatment of sunburn

- Removal from sun.

- Cool soaks.

- Aloe.

- Consider ibuprofen for pain relief.

- Hydration. (See pg. 76)

Sun Poisoning: A syndrome combining dehydration with excessive UV exposure.

Signs and symptoms

- Weakness, fever, nausea, vomiting, loss of appetite.

Treatment

- Remove from sun/heat.

- Cool soaks.

- Hydration.

Chemical Burns

Treatment

1. Remove contaminant – brush off of skin. Remove contaminated clothing and flush area with **copious** amounts of water. Be aware to not flush chemical onto non-injured areas, especially to eyes, nose, mouth, etc.

2. For plastics and tar, cool with large amounts of water. Do not peel off.

Electrical Burns (Lightning in Particular)

Treatment

1. Do not touch the patient unless electricity is off (lightning-strike patients are not electrically "hot" after a strike. Touching them will not shock you). Be alert for repeat lightning strikes.

2. Assess and stabilize the airway.

3. Aggressive CPR if patient is pulseless. These patients respond well to resuscitative efforts.

4. Suspect other trauma, especially c-spine.

Evacuation Criteria for Burns

1. **Rapid evacuation** for partial thickness burns greater than 9% BSA.
2. **Rapid evacuation** for any airway burn involving:
   - Charring or singed hair around the nose or mouth
   - Hoarse voice or wheezing
   - Grey-black productive cough
   - Swelling around the mouth or neck
   - Shortness of breath
   - Rapid respiratory rate
3. **Evacuate** any full-thickness burn.
   - Rapid evacuation for full-thickness burns greater than 1% BSA.
4. **Evacuate** any partial-thickness burns involving:
   - Face, eyes, neck, chest, hands/feet, genitalia.
   - Associated fractures.
   - Burn around the circumference of an extremity ("circumferential").
   - Greater than 1% body surface area (or greater than palm size).
5. *Consider* evacuation for blistering sunburns or signs and symptoms of sun poisoning.

Musculoskeletal Trauma

Background

PREVALENCE: Regardless of the activity, sprains, strains and fractures are among the most common backcountry injuries. Together, these injuries probably delay or stop more outdoor adventures than any other injury type. Their prevention, assessment, and proper treatment should be priorities for all wilderness medicine providers.

DEFINITIONS:

Strain: Inflammation or overuse injury to a tendon, a structure connecting muscle to bone, or muscle.

Sprain: A tear (complete or partial) of a ligament, a structure connecting bone to bone.

Fracture: A break (complete or partial) in a bone. Fractures are classified as **open** (break in the skin at fracture site) **or closed** (skin at fracture site is still intact).

Dislocation: An injury in which normal articulation of a joint is disrupted due to displacement of one of the articulating bones. Many are associated with fractures.

Contusion: Bruising with no break in the skin. Mechanisms of injury include a direct or crushing force.

Signs and Symptoms

- The pain from a contusion may be more or less than a fracture. If in doubt, treat the injury as a fracture.
- These types of injuries swell, sometimes far more than what you might expect. Bruising a bone near a joint may cause significant inflammation of the joint.

Treatment

First 48 Hours: Rest, ice (20-30 minutes every 2 hours), compression, elevation. Ice should not be directly applied to the skin.

48-72 Hours: Warm packs 2-3 times daily for 15-20 minutes, compression, pain-free activity.

Consider ibuprofen or other non-steroidal anti-inflammatory drugs (NSAIDs). Be sure to ask if there are allergies to recommended medication.

Assessment for Orthopedic Injuries

Begin by gathering information about the incident from the scene, the patient, and any bystanders:

1. **Mechanism of Injury** – Find out what exactly happened. How far was the fall? What did the person land on? What hole did the patient step into? Has he or she tried to stand or use the injured extremity? Was the patient unable to bear weight or to use extremity?
2. **Pertinent Patient History** – Ask if the person has a history of this type of injury. Ask the patient what they heard or felt at the time of the injury.
3. **General Impression of the Patient** – Pay attention to the position of limb, amount of blood loss, the presence of open wounds and any spontaneous movement of extremity. Ask if the patient can bear weight.

NOTE: Always investigate the possibility of an underlying medical issue preceding the fall/injury.

Physical Exam

1. Assess the **location** of the injury.
2. Expose the area. Assess the **skin** for **color, temperature, and moisture (SCTM)** as well as the presence of any angulations, swelling, and open wounds.
3. **Compare** both sides of the body (bilateral symmetry) looking for swelling, bruising, or deformity on the injured side compared to the non-injured side.
4. Check distal **circulation** (pulses and capillary refill), **sensation**, and **movement (CSM).**
5. Feel for crepitus, tenderness, and stability of long bones.
6. Assess range of motion by asking the patient to move the injured area, *as long as this does not cause pain* (active movement). Assess passive range of motion by gently moving the limb yourself. **Stop** if pain increases or resistance is met. Avoid passively moving a limb if the patient refuses to move it.

Sprains and Strains

	STRAINS	SPRAINS	FRACTURES	DISLOCATIONS
Mechanism of Injury	Over time or sudden, due to improper technique	Sudden, jarring, twisting	Sudden, associated with impact or force	Sudden, indirect or direct force or impact on a joint
Patient History	Often has history	May have history	Probably no history	Often has history
Signs & Symptoms	Swelling, redness, noises and pain associated with activity that caused strain	Swelling, pain, bruising discoloration, decreased/inability to bear weight, "popping sound"	Swelling, pain, bruising, point tenderness, crepitus, angulation, deformity, inability to bear weight, may be open	Deformity at joint, loss of symmetry, abnormal shape, lack of obvious angulation, loss of joint function
Treatment	RICES	RICES	RICES, consider reduction if severely angulated or CMS is compromised	Splint or reduce depending upon distal CSM, location, relationship to patient, assessment skills
Prevention	Warm-up Hydrate Proper conditioning/ training	Warm-up Good boots Proper conditioning/ training	Remain within skill level	Proper conditioning/training Proper form and technique

Sprains and Strains Treatment

RICES – Rest, Ice, Compression, Elevation and Stabilization

RICES are generally applied when the injury appears relatively minor and the patient can tolerate some movement. Use on sprains and strains to reduce and prevent excessive swelling.

1. **REST** - Do not use the extremity for approximately 24-48 hours, if possible, or until the patient:
   - Can bear weight without pain **and**
   - Has decreased swelling around the injury.

2. **ICE/ IBUPROFEN (NSAID)** - Apply cold to injury for 10 minutes on/ 10 off, for the first 24-48 hours after injury. Consider ibuprofen or other Non-Steroidal Anti-Inflammatory Drug (NSAID). As always, ask the patient about allergies or other adverse reactions that they have had to these medications. Consider combining NSAIDs with acetaminophen (Tylenol/ Paracetamol) for greater pain relief.

3. **COMPRESSION** - Wrap the injury with a compression wrap (e.g., ACE® wrap) snugly, but not tightly, beginning distally and wrapping proximally.

4. **ELEVATION** - Elevate the extremity above the heart to reduce swelling.

5. **STABILIZATION** - Support the extremity after 24-48 hours of rest (if you have the luxury to wait that long). Support the extremity with a splint or tape if the patient can bear weight without pain and if swelling is reduced.

NOTE: **Splinting** or otherwise immobilizing the joint or extremity is often the best option if the injury appears to be more severe, the injury site is unstable, and/or the joint or extremity is not functional.

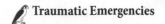

> ## Critical Thinking for Orthopedic Injuries
>
> Extremity injuries hurt, and they may pose significant evacuation challenges, putting an entire group at risk. A well-constructed splint or brace will both decrease the pain and maintain circulation and neurologic function. Splints can make the difference between a self-evacuation and an extended, complicated rescue. Conversely, improper treatment will often cause more pain and can result in permanent damage. Be thorough in your assessment and conservative in your actions. It would be nice to distinguish between sprains, strains, fractures, contusions, and dislocations because the treatment for each differs to some degree; **however, a definitive diagnosis is often not possible, *and much good can still be done without a diagnosis.***

Splinting

Background

Splinting is the process of immobilizing bones and/or joints with suspected fractures, dislocations, severe sprains and/ or significant pain. Good splints reduce unintentional and painful motion, support injured areas and accommodate swelling. Injuries requiring splints generally require evacuation.

Splinting Guidelines:

1. Keep them Simple

- Complicated splints tend to fall apart. Splints do not need to be complex or difficult to remember how to build. Keep in mind patients will be moving and it will need adjusted. Making it simple will allow you to re-adjust while keeping the splint comfortable for the patient.

2. Check Before and After

- Check distal CSM of the extremity before applying the splint. Once you have applied a splint, you must re-check distal CSM and compare.

3. Immobilize Above and Below

- A splint should immobilize the joints above and below the injury. If it is a joint injury, immobilize the long bones above and below the injury.

4. Avoid the Void

- Pad well, filling voids with foam or other soft material like clothing.

5. Position of Function

- Splint extremities in a natural position. For example, splints for the hand should leave the fingers curled inward.

Fractures

Background

DEFINITION: Fractures are breaks (complete or partial) in a bone. Fractures are classified as **open** (break in the skin at fracture site) **or closed** (skin at fracture site is still intact).

DETAILS: Every fracture will have its own set of special circumstances and challenges in the backcountry. Some are life-threatening, while most are not. Prevention, good assessment, and safe evacuation are the goals.

Upper Extremity Injuries

1. Clavicle

A fracture of the clavicle (collarbone) may result from a fall onto an outstretched arm (indirect force) or from a direct impact with an object. Be alert for signs of difficulty breathing; the fracture could have damaged the underlying lung. Be alert for signs of internal bleeding. The fracture could have injured the subclavian artery. Assess the upper extremity for neurologic abnormalities. The fracture could have injured the brachial plexus nerves.

SPLINTING: Immobilization can be achieved by a simple sling and swathe.

2. Humerus

Direct or indirect force to the upper arm may fracture the humerus.

SPLINTING: Immobilize with rigid support from the shoulder to the elbow plus a sling and swathe.

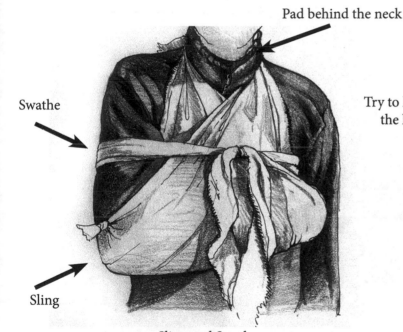

Pad behind the neck

Swathe

Sling

Sling and Swathe

Try to keep the hand above
the level of the elbow.

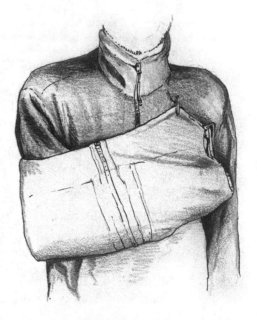

Shirt Sling
Safety-pinned in Place

3. Forearm (Radius, Ulna, Elbow or Wrist)

Numerous types of forearm/wrist fractures may result from falls onto hands, depending on the position of the appendage and the amount and location of force. **Never forcefully realign or reduce angulated forearm fractures.**

SPLINTING: Immobilize forearm injuries from elbow to hand. If the elbow is injured, the humerus should also be splinted. Mold the splint on the uninjured arm. Splint the forearm with a rigid support (SAM® splint), then place something (e.g., gauze roll or sock) in the patient's hand to maintain a *position of function.* Pad the splint and fill in all the spaces. Complete immobilization with a sling and swathe.

4. Fingers and Toes

SPLINTING: A fractured finger or toe may be taped to an adjacent finger (buddy splint) for support, or a more elaborate splint may be constructed with a small rigid support.

Lower Extremity Injuries

1. Tibia/Fibula

Sometimes known as a "boot-top" fracture, these injuries may result from foot or lower leg entrapment, twisting or direct/indirect force to the lower leg.

SPLINTING: Numerous materials may be improvised to immobilize the lower leg: ski poles, SAM® splints, backpack stays, foam sleeping pads, etc. Depending on patient comfort, flex the knee slightly and place a pad in the void under the knee.

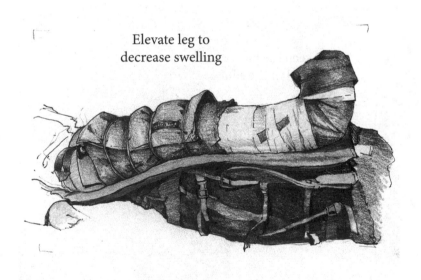

Elevate leg to decrease swelling

Splint of tibia/fibula

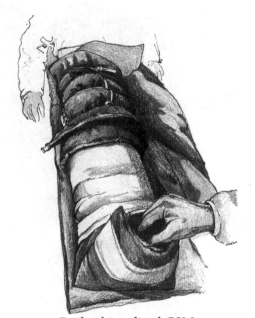

Rechecking distal CSM

2. Foot/Ankle

Falls onto the feet may fracture one or many of the bones in the feet. Likewise, a sudden twisting force may break an ankle.

SPLINTING: Immobilization can be achieved easily with a foam sleeping pad or Crazy Creek™ chair. SAM® splints are also useful. Consider securing the legs together to prevent foot rotation.

Fractures with Special Considerations

Angulated Fractures

DEFINITION:

Angulated fracture: A fracture that is no longer in anatomical position or out of natural alignment.

Realignment: A gentle realignment (brought back to an in-line, natural position) of a long bone using slight traction (steady, light pull distally).

RISKS:

Angulated fractures pose significant risk to the patient and a challenge to the provider. An angulation may disrupt circulation and impinge nerves; with time, swelling can further inhibit CSM if the injury is left misaligned. Effective splinting is difficult to achieve and positioning during evacuation is problematic. However, damage can occur during realignment. The nerves and vessels are at some risk of becoming entrapped or torn during its reduction or realignment. Before acting, prudent providers must consider difficulty of evacuation, their relationship to the patient, relevant protocols and regulations, and their familiarity with the procedure.

1. **In general, it is wise to attempt realignment if:**
   - You are more than 2 hours from care _and_
   - The extremity is unstable, moves independently, and is easily straightened _and_
   - The angulation precludes stable splinting for evacuation _and_
   - There is diminished distal CSM.

2. **Do NOT realign if:**
   - You meet resistance while moving the extremity _or_
   - There is any sudden increase in pain during realignment. Some pain is expected.

3. **In addition, this decision is easier if:**
   - The patient is not your client, but rather a friend or family member
   - The patient is not a minor (adults can make informed decisions)
   - The procedure is in accordance with local regulations
   - You have physician or organizational protocols to perform the procedure

Open Fractures

DEFINITION:

Any fracture with an open break in the skin near the site of the fracture, often the result of bone ends breaking through the skin and tissue. Bone may be visible or may retract into the wound.

RISKS:

An open fracture is contaminated and at high risk for complicated infection. Bleeding may occur from the wound as well as from the marrow of the bone.

Treatment

1. Perform early, high pressure (6-12 psi) irrigation with 1-3 liters of potable water.
2. Apply moistened sterile dressings to open wounds and exposed bone; change dressing every 24 hours.
3. If concurrent angulation exists, irrigate before attempting realignment.
4. Splint with "window" to wound site.

Evacuation Criteria for Fractures

1. **Rapid evacuation** of all open fractures.
2. **Rapid evacuation** for all fractures that result in compromised or loss of distal CSM.
3. **Evacuate** all suspected fractures.

Pelvic Fractures

DEFINITION: A fracture of the pelvic girdle. Pelvic fractures result from high-force impacts directly to the pelvic ring. Fractures typically occur in more than one place on the pelvis.

RISKS: Pelvic fractures are always emergencies and should be addressed during the primary survey. (See page 38)

Signs and Symptoms

- Pelvic fractures are often extremely painful. Much of the pain is due to instability.
- Pelvic instability
- Pelvic girdle crepitus
- Possible signs of shock

Treatment

1. Anticipate and treat for shock.

2. Keep the patient warm.

3. Minimize rolling the patient or further manipulation of the pelvic region.

4. Stabilize the pelvis utilizing a manufactured or improvised pelvic wrap.

   - Rotate feet to forward position. Pad space between the legs and buddy splint legs together.
   - Apply pelvic wrap at the level of the greater trochanters (level with the groin).
   - Improvised pelvic wraps can be constructed from backpack hip belts, folded air mattresses (Therm-a-rest™), SAM splints and tourniquet, coats or other material, or cut pants.
   - Position and secure the patient to a litter.
   - Provide spinal motion restriction (SMR), when indicated.

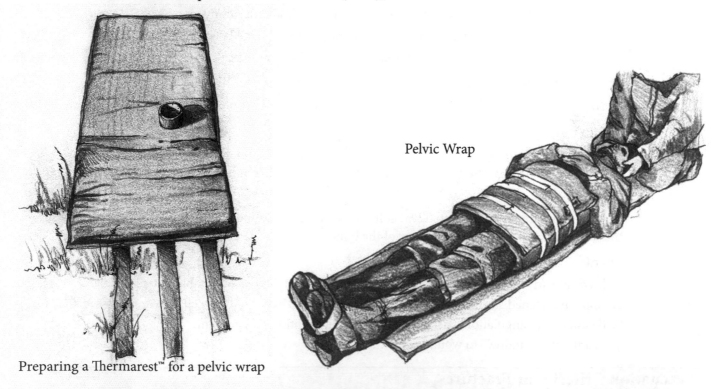

Pelvic Wrap

Preparing a Thermarest™ for a pelvic wrap

Evacuation Criteria for Suspected Pelvic Fractures

Rapid evacuation for all suspected pelvic fractures.

Aerie Backcountry Medicine © 14th Edition

Femur Fractures

CAUSES: Femur fractures usually require a high-impact force or significant MOI.

RISKS: Large arteries and veins traverse the upper leg, making fractures to this area particularly prone to significant bleeding. The space within an adult's upper leg is capable of holding about two liters of blood. In addition, because of the forces required to fracture a femur, providers should consider the possibility of spinal trauma. Immediate management of these injuries is required to reduce additional damage and minimize pain. Applying an improvised traction device in a wilderness setting, however, is controversial. Applied improperly, an improvised traction device can harm both injured and previously uninjured tissue. In most cases, a simple, well-constructed splint that reduces motion, but does NOT pull traction, is the most practical treatment option.

Signs and Symptoms

- Pain
- Swelling and/or discoloration of thigh
- Deformity of femur
- Point tenderness in mid-shaft region of femur
- External rotation and shortening of the injured leg
- Anticipate and watch for shock.

Treatment

- **ABCDEs** – Keep the patient warm.
- **Manual stabilization** of the femur. Hold the lower leg immobile until a splint is made.
- Check distal **CSM** of injured leg.
- **Splint in place**. Support the ankle and foot for patient comfort.
- Assess for **shock** and treat accordingly.

Evacuation Criteria

Rapid evacuation for all suspected femur fractures.

Dislocations

CAUSES: Strong forces directed on a joint or its surrounding structures are capable of causing the joint to dislocate. A common mechanism is that of a kayaker performing a high-brace in which one arm is raised and externally rotated. The shallow ball-and-socket joint at the shoulder is disrupted as the head of the humerus is levered out of position.

Specific Dislocations

1. Shoulder

Anterior: >90% of shoulder injuries will dislocate anteriorly. The head of the humerus will displace anterior to shoulder joint and can often be seen or felt in the axilla (armpit).

Posterior: The head of the humerus lies posterior to shoulder joint (rare and usually associated with fractures).

DO NOT reduce posterior dislocations. Splint in place and evacuate.

Signs and Symptoms of an <u>Anterior</u> Shoulder Dislocation

- The classic presentation for an anterior dislocation is with a patient holding the affected arm down and **away** from the body. The patient will be most likely be unable to touch his elbow to his waist. This is very different from other arm or shoulder injuries, where the patient self-splints the arm by holding it directly against the body.

- The upper arm loses its "rounded-off" edge under the deltoid muscle and instead looks "squared-off" at the lateral margin of the scapula. (Remember, though, that this is not always straightforward.)

- If the dislocation was caused by direct force or significant MOI where a fracture cannot be ruled out, **DO NOT reduce. Instead, splint in place and evacuate.**

Treatment of an <u>Anterior</u> Shoulder Dislocation

- Check distal CSM.

- Reduce passively.

  1. **Seated reduction** – Have the patient sit with knees flexed to chest (upright fetal position) and arms wrapped around knees. The patient then leans back causing their own body weight to fatigue the muscles and allow the joint to reduce.

  2. **Hanging reduction** – Place the patient prone on a flat surface that is high enough to allow the arm to hang straight down. Suspend 5-10 pounds of weight by the wrist. Attach water bottles, a pot of water or other weight to a padded sling on the wrist (1 liter of water weighs about 2 pounds). As the shoulder muscles fatigue, the joint should reduce back into position. It may take up to 45 minutes for this to work. To aid this reduction technique, consider a scapular massage.

- Re-check distal CSM.

- Splint the arm with a sling and swathe.

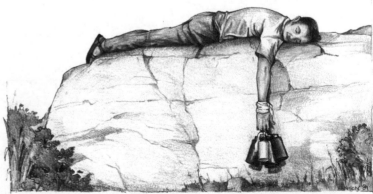

Hanging Reduction

2. Finger

Signs and Symptoms

- A phalange (finger bone) of the finger is forced out of position.
- Obvious deformity occurs.
- The joint is locked into position.

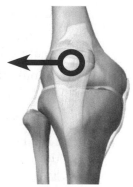

Do not reduce thumb joints.

Only consider reducing the two distal most joints.

Treatment

- With one hand, apply gentle traction to the distal portion of the finger and, with the other hand, push the dislocated end back into place.
- Tape it to a neighboring finger for a few days to prevent re-injury.

3. Knee Cap (Patella)

Signs and Symptoms

- The patella, a bone within the patellar tendon of the quadriceps muscle, can become dislocated from its normally flat position on the knee joint.
- The deformity can be obvious with thin patients, but more difficult with obese or extremely muscular patients.
- The patient will not want to straighten the knee joint.

The patella is often dislocated laterally towards the fibula (outside).

Treatment

- Check distal CSM.
- The patient should lie supine, with the injured leg raised.
- Slowly straighten the knee while guiding the patella back into position.
- Re-check CSM.
- May need to be splinted.

Critical Thinking and Evacuation Criteria for Dislocations

Reduction of a dislocation is often tricky. You may cause further harm if you act hastily. However, leaving a joint dislocated for many hours will also cause damage. This decision should further be influenced by your relationship with the patient, your familiarity with the assessment and the procedure, local regulations, and your institutional protocols, if any. Anyone who informs you that the assessment of dislocations is straightforward or that the treatment is without risk is misinformed.

1. If in the backcountry, you *may* choose to attempt reduction if:
   - MOI, detailed assessment, and patient history do not suggest a fracture.
   - You are more than two hours from definitive care.
   - The patient's injury is causing a disruption to distal circulation, sensation and/ or motion.
   - *NOTE*: This is also dependent upon your protocols, laws, and your relationship with the patient.
2. If reduction techniques cause a severe, unexplained increase in pain, or the reduction takes more than one hour, STOP, splint, and **evacuate**.
3. If you decide against reduction, splint (creatively) in the position of comfort and **evacuate** the patient. Continually re-assess the injury site and distal CSM function.
4. If the dislocation is open (broke the skin), splint and immobilize the extremity for **evacuation**.

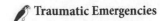

Evacuation Decisions

Background

Backcountry evacuations are time-consuming and often difficult operations. The complexity, time commitment and number of people required for an evacuation is variable. In ideal conditions, a carried litter evacuation might move about 1 mile per hour and require a team of 15-20 people. Technical terrain requires more training, skills and specialized equipment. Additionally, weather, distance, and time of day can change the difficulty and requirements of an evacuation. Recognizing the difference between emergent and non-emergent evacuations will determine the most appropriate type of evacuation and strategies.

BACKCOUNTRY EVACUATION CONSIDERATIONS:

- Is the situation emergent or non-emergent?
    - Can the patient be stabilized or is their condition deteriorating?
- Does this situation require additional resources or professional rescue teams?
- Is an improvised evacuation technique, such as an improvised litter, practical, or does the situation require a professional rescue team and manufactured equipment?
- Should the rescuers hike at night or wait until morning?
    - Ensure that all members of the rescue team are equipped to spend the night out.
    - Night operations involve additional risks to rescue personnel and aircraft.
- Is it possible to have relief personnel?
- Can the mission be accomplished without rescue personnel traveling alone?

EVACUATION TYPES:

The differences in patients needs, weather considerations, accessibility, terrain, and rescuer safety determine the type of evacuation and the techniques to employ during an evacuation.

1. **Locate/Simple Subject Assist** - A simple locate-and-assist evacuation is suitable for subjects that are lost or in need of evacuation from the field but still able to travel under their own power over easily-managed terrain. Often, this can be accomplished with fewer people and might simply be walking a subject to a trailhead.

2. **Simple Carry/Litter Evacuation** - For patients that have a musculoskeletal or medical injury that prevents them from evacuating under their own power. A litter carry will also be employed for patients that require spinal motion restriction. Consider the distance for a litter evacuation. Shorter distances and moderate to easily managed terrain. Often the simple litter carry can be in the form of an improvised litter construction and carried out, one-wheeled Litter, toboggan, or litter attachment for motorized transport for this type of evacuation. Although the terrain may be relatively easy, a carried litter evacuation will limit the type of medical treatments that can be accomplished or sustained throughout the evacuation.

3. **Technical Litter Evacuation** - The technical litter evacuation is used for patients that require litter evacuation out of high-angle terrain. Typically high-angle terrain is >20 degrees to vertical. Challenging terrain requires specialized technical skills and equipment to properly execute a safe patient evacuation. This includes rope systems, technical equipment, and high-angle training and techniques. The technical evacuation will limit medical treatments that can be provided or sustained during these operations.

4. **Helicopter Evacuations** - There are two distinct types of helicopter evacuations, SAR and air-ambulance. Both operations come with an added set of considerations. Proper helicopter safety and functional organization of team resources will ensure the smooth integration of helicopter operations.

1. Search and rescue (SAR) helicopter transport and short haul/hoist helicopter evacuations: Using the helicopter to assist in evacuating the subject from challenging terrain or a place where there is no landing zone. SAR helicopter transport can also be used for a subject that needs extrication to a trailhead, ground ambulance, or air ambulance.
2. Air ambulance helicopter: Often staffed with professional care providers, an air ambulance is used for critical and unstable patients requiring advanced care or rapid transport to a definitive care facility. Any patient requiring rapid evacuation should be considered for air ambulance transport.

EVACUATION ORGANIZATION:

The organization of an evacuation can greatly affect the outcome. Clearly defining roles and responsibilities increases the effectiveness of an evacuation and increases mission success. There are five clearly defined leadership positions to consider when organizing an evacuation of any kind.

1. **Site Commander**: The site commander is in charge of the scene. Often they are the highest qualified or predetermined as the group leader. In a formal SAR response, the site commander will be answering to an overall incident commander. The site commander is responsible for deciding on the method for evacuation as well as assigning team members roles and responsibilities. The site commander will also direct efforts during the evacuation.
2. **Patent care/attendant**: The attendant is responsible for all patient care throughout the evacuation. Along with stabilization and medical intervention, the attendant acts as a communication vector and patient advocate. The attendant remains with the patient until there is a clear patient handoff, with all questions answered to a new attendant or transporting agency.
3. **Communication**: The communications personnel are responsible for developing an effective communication plan and means of communication between all personnel.
4. **Rigging**: Rigging personnel are responsible for the technical systems and equipment needed for low and high-angle rescues. Rigging personnel might also be responsible for the operation of litter evacuation systems.
5. **Safety**: A dedicated person for safety consideration helps ensure the safe and smooth operation of an evacuation. They are responsible for overall operational safety as well as individual rescuer safety during an evacuation.

Litters for Patient Evacuation

TARP OR BLANKET LITTER:

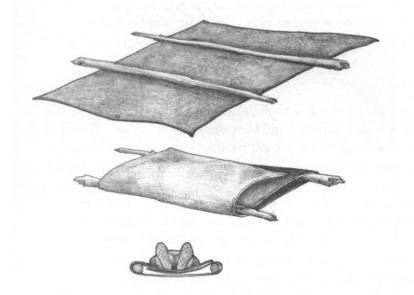

- The **tarp or blanket litter** is a very effective device for moving patients short distances. It is quickly and easily made from materials on-hand.

ROPE LITTER:

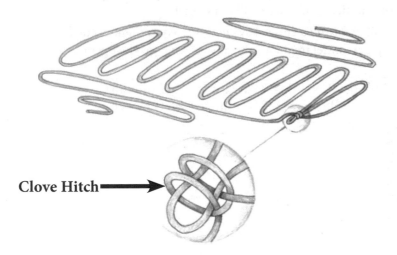

Clove Hitch →

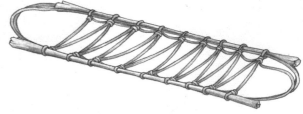

- A **rope litter** can be made with 75-150 feet (23-45 meters) of rope, which may be spliced together.
- With rigid stays and pads and/or packs; it can provide spinal protection. Without these, it is best used for patients without spinal injuries.
- Rope litters take time to construct and require practice.
- Rope litters are durable and easy to carry.

Critical Thinking for Litters and Evacuation:

- Anyone who has ever carried a patient on a litter knows the work, personnel needed, danger (for the rescuers and the patient), equipment, and time involved. Calling for outside help is usually necessary.
- Although we *can* construct litters, for the above reasons it is usually not prudent to use them for carrying our patients very far without additional help.
- However, litters are invaluable for moving a patient to camp, out of danger, or to a landing zone. In addition, they can make it possible for one provider to roll a patient to clear their airway repeatedly while waiting for outside help.
- Like most skills learned, those of litter construction need to account for the specifics of the emergency.

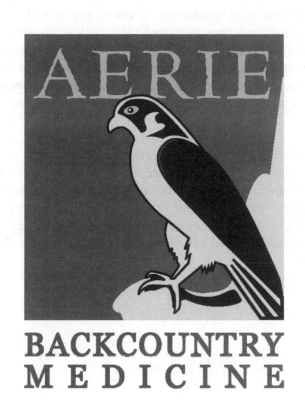

Section Five:
Medical Emergencies

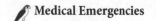

Medical Emergencies

Background

DEFINITION: Medical emergencies are typically defined as physiological problems not resulting from external, physical trauma. They include everything from constipation to heart attacks, and may also result from a psychological rather than physiological crisis. As such, medical emergencies cause any combination of pain, weakness and altered levels of consciousness.

DECISION-MAKING: Do you want to make this as simple as possible? Throughout your assessment, and particularly when making evacuation decisions, think "sick or not sick" rather than, for example "appendicitis or ectopic pregnancy". It is often difficult and sometimes impossible to know what is causing a patient's pain, weakness, or altered mental status. You should be well-versed on both the more common, benign problems, and the less common, truly life-threatening medical problems. In the end, use your best judgment. Some of the best decisions are based on the assessment that a person simply looks ill.

PREVENTION: There are several ways to prevent medical emergencies. Whenever possible, maintain hygiene, remain well-hydrated, well-fed, well-rested, and properly-clothed. Become informed about your backcountry partners' and clients' health histories. Learn the terrain, respect the wildlife, and pay attention to the weather. Finally, keep your guard up when your energy is down, especially at the end of the day. Create a life routine that supports a healthy mind and body. Of course, injuries and illnesses occur to even the best prepared. However, efforts toward prevention will also benefit you when unexpected events occur.

Cardiac Emergencies

Background

790,000 Americans experience myocardial infarction every year. Chest discomfort may result from muscle strains or gastrointestinal problems such as heartburn. These are usually not an emergency; however, chest pain of a cardiac origin **is** an emergency. These patients often have a history of heart disease and tend to look sick.

Risk Factors

1. Cardiac history
2. High blood pressure
3. Smoking
4. High cholesterol
5. Family history
6. Male or post-menopausal female
7. Obese or significantly overweight
8. Inactive
9. Diabetes

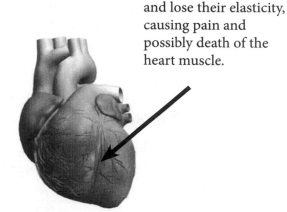

These are the coronary arteries that clog, spasm, and lose their elasticity, causing pain and possibly death of the heart muscle.

Precipitating Factors

1. Exercise/exertion
2. Anxiety/fear
3. May have no recognizable precipitating factors

Signs and Symptoms

1. Chest discomfort, squeezing or pain that is typically not affected by body position, breathing, or palpation of the chest wall. Discomfort and pain are less common in women than men.
2. Pain that radiates into the arm or jaw or between the shoulder blades
3. Shortness of breath ⎫
4. Nausea, vomiting ⎪
5. Sweating ⎬ This patient looks sick
6. Pale Skin ⎪
7. Weakness, dizziness ⎭
8. Anxiety/fear/denial
9. Syncope (fainting), near syncope

Treatment

1. Reduce patient activity and anxiety.
2. Allow patient to maintain a position of comfort.
3. Consider suggesting the patient take 324 mg of chewable, non-coated aspirin.
4. Evacuate the patient with the least amount of movement/exertion possible.
5. Consider air evacuation for suspected heart attack.
6. Prepare for the possible cardiac arrest requiring CPR, an AED, additional personnel, etc.

Critical Thinking and Evacuation Criteria for Cardiac Emergencies

The pain and discomfort of a heart attack is generally different from musculoskeletal pain. In your assessment of a patient with chest pain, pay close attention to the symptoms described and the patient history. It may be very difficult to determine the cause of the pain. Consider everything you can learn about the patient and err on the side of caution.

- **Rapid evacuation** if a cardiac cause of the discomfort is suspected.

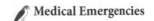

Dehydration

Background

CAUSES: Blood is mostly water. Any condition that impairs water intake (nausea, vomiting) or increases water output (excessive sweating, diarrhea, bleeding, burns) reduces blood, interstitial (fluid around tissue and cells), and cellular (fluid within the cell) volume, and impairs the function of all body systems. Dehydration is a significant killer throughout the world. It is a great masquerader, resembling, if not exacerbating, other illnesses and injuries including hypothermia, head injuries, low blood sugar, and high altitude illnesses.

PREVENTION: Like so much in medicine, preventing dehydration is often easier than treating it. Work vigilantly to maintain hydration by drinking often (4-6 liters a day in a hot environment). Do yourself a huge hydration favor and keep feces out of your food and water at all costs. Some general guidelines for drinking water are as follows: drink 1 liter of water 1 to 2 hours before activity begins, then about 1 liter of water for every hour of activity or about 1 to 2 liters per mile hiked. Do not drink more than 10 liters in 24 hours. Schedule frequent rest and hydration stops, maintain good nutrition, and make water palatable. Maintain your own hydration, while watching your partners closely for good habits.

Signs and Symptoms

1. Fatigue
2. Confusion (poor decision making)
3. Irritability
4. Headache (HA)
5. Nausea, vomiting (N/V)
6. Infrequent, yellow urine
7. Dry mucosa (lips, eyes)
8. Poor skin elasticity
9. Dizziness, particularly when suddenly standing up
10. Syncope or near syncope
11. Signs and symptoms of shock

Oral Rehydration Salt Recipe

The World Health Organization recommends:

- In one liter of water, add
- 3.5 g NaCl (sodium chloride/ table salt)
- 1.5 g KCl (potassium chloride/ dietary salt)
- 2.5 g NaHCO3 (sodium bicarbonate/ baking soda)
- 20 g glucose (table sugar)

Which roughly corresponds to:

- 1 liter of water
- ½ teaspoon table salt
- ¼ teaspoon dietary salt
- ½ teaspoon baking soda
- 3 tablespoons of sugar

Treatment

1. Reduce activity.
2. If in a sunny and hot environment, cool with evaporation and shade.
3. Slowly rehydrate as patient can tolerate, starting with about 200 ml/hr.
   - Have patient drink enough to maintain good urine output and avoid vomiting.
4. Consider need for electrolyte replacement (particularly for vomiting/diarrhea).
5. Maintain nutritional needs with simple foods easily-tolerated by patient.

Critical Thinking and Evacuation Criteria for Dehydration

Dehydration is serious when it makes a person feel weak and look sick. In small children, dehydration can be life threatening within the first few hours of diarrhea, nausea and vomiting. With adults, this process takes longer, but, in the end, the sicker looking and more fatigued they get, the more serious is the problem.

- **Evacuate** if you are unable to rehydrate a patient over 24-48 hours.
- **Evacuate** if S/S of shock are present.

Abdominal Medical Emergencies

"Common Things Are Common"

Background

CAUSES: Complaints of "stomach" or abdominal pain are frequent and usually not life threatening. Most result from changes in diet or intestinal parasites introduced from poor campsite/cooking hygiene or contaminated water. These are easily prevented, often self-correcting, and typically treated with time, simple diet, and clean water. In contrast, abdominal issues resulting in severe pain, infection, or blood loss can be life-threatening and require prompt evacuation.

Assessment

1. **ABCDEs**

2. **SAMPLE/OPQRST**

   - Obtain a thorough history. Clues to the underlying cause of discomfort may come from the questions you ask.

3. **Physical Exam**

   - **Overall**:

     How does the patient *look*? Sick/ not sick; skin color, temperature and moisture conditions, etc.
     What is the patient *doing*? Guarding, strange positions of comfort, vomiting, etc.

   - **Abdomen**:

     Look for redness, bruising, distention or other abnormalities.
     Feel for tenderness, rigidity, distention, rebound pain, and temperature. **Palpate** each of the four quadrants of the abdomen.

4. **Vital Signs**

   - Assess level of responsiveness (LOR).

   - Assess heart rate, rhythm and quality (HR).

   - Assess respiratory rate, rhythm, and quality (RR).

Critical Thinking and Evacuation Criteria for Abdominal Emergencies

Differentiating between abdominal illnesses that are life threats and those that are not is difficult and rarely results in a definitive field diagnosis. For example, it is less common to know that a patient has appendicitis than it is to recognize that the patient looks quite ill and has signs and symptoms consistent with serious illness, of which appendicitis is a possibility. It is important, therefore, to understand the common causes of abdominal discomfort, both benign and life-threatening. It is particularly important to have some criteria with which you will decide whether a particular pain or discomfort warrants evacuation.

1. **Evacuate** abdominal pain/discomfort following significant abdominal trauma.
2. **Evacuate** significant abdominal pain/discomfort lasting greater than 24 hours.
3. **Evacuate** abdominal pain/discomfort that precludes or greatly limits walking, moving, or eating.
4. **Evacuate** abdominal pain/discomfort associated with the inability to drink or retain fluids for more than 24 hours.
5. **Evacuate** abdominal pain/discomfort with the possibility of pregnancy.
6. **Evacuate** abdominal pain/discomfort with a rigid or distended abdomen.
7. **Evacuate** abdominal pain/discomfort with fever.
8. **Evacuate** abdominal pain/discomfort with signs and symptoms of shock.

PROBLEM/ CONDITION	SIGNS AND SYMPTOMS	TREATMENT	PREVENTION
Nausea/ Vomiting	Look for blood Dehydration Fever possible	Position of comfort Clear fluids, sports drinks in small amounts at first, if tolerated for 12 hours, try simple foods Rest	Good hygiene
Constipation/ Fecal Impaction	Very individual-dependent Lack of bowel movements (defined as fewer than 3 bowel movements/ week) Diffuse cramps and/or abdominal pain Urge to defecate	Hydration Caffeine, fruit Consider laxatives	Maintain hydration Monitor defecation frequency Maintain good defecation environment (*some people do not want to poop in a hole*)
Diarrhea	Frequent, watery stools; blood, pain, fever Look for dehydration	Oral Rehydration Salt (ORS) Clear fluids and sports drinks for 24 hrs, then consider mild foods Limit caffeine Consider Imodium® or Lomotil™ if persistent and no fever Bismuth (Pepto-Bismol™)	Good hygiene Careful eating habits Good food sharing practices Water treatment
Appendicitis	Looks sick. Pain begins in the center of the abdomen, moves to RLQ, becomes more constant, more severe N/V, diarrhea, low-grade fever, rebound pain, S/S infection, lack of appetite is common, sudden decrease in pain could mean rupture Fetal position often assumed	Position of comfort Consider early evacuation	
Kidney Stones	Often the worst pain ever felt by patient Flank to anterior pain in abdomen (near kidney region to the groin) Often intense pain with urination >2/3 are males, with a previous history	Position of comfort Fluids Treat dehydration	Hydration For some people, diet
Bleeding	Melena (dark, digested blood in stools) Bloody vomit (looks like used coffee grounds) Rigid abdomen sometimes seen	Position of comfort Clear liquids only Early evacuation Consider antibiotics for traveler's diarrhea	Clean food and water to prevent infections
Intestinal Parasites/Giardia/ Cryptosporidium	Bloating (7-21 days following exposure) Pain, diarrhea, cramps, sulfuric smell, and flatulence	Rest Consider antibiotics Hydrate	Treat your water Good camp hygiene
Urinary Tract Infection	Frequent, painful, and/or non- productive urination May have blood	Hydrate Consider antibiotics Monitor for worsening S/S	Good hygiene, diet, hydration
Ectopic Pregnancy	First trimester pregnancy Abdominal pain, vaginal bleeding Shock History of infections, surgeries, STDs	Position of comfort Immediate evacuation	

Allergic Reactions and Anaphylaxis

Background

EPIDEMIOLOGY: Although reports of nonfatal anaphylaxis are relatively common, it is an uncommon cause of death. The actual rate of anaphylaxis is difficult to ascertain, as it is underreported. The leading cause of fatal anaphylaxis is allergic reaction to drug administration, the majority of which occur in healthcare facilities. Food allergies and insect stings make up the majority of remaining fatal cases.

PREVENTION: Prevention centers around minimizing the chance of exposure in those with known allergies. For organized activities this begins with appropriate medical screening of participants to identify those with known allergies and to assure that appropriate medications are available. Less formally, it can include knowing your partner or team member's medical histories, including allergies, and knowing where they keep medications for their treatment. Consider not allowing a particular food on a backcountry trip if someone within your party has a known allergy to that food.

ANATOMY AND PHYSIOLOGY: An allergic reaction is the body's response to an allergen or antigen, such as wasp venom. A body develops antibodies to particular allergens based on exposure and immunological predisposition. At some future exposure to the antigen (not necessarily the very next), the body's immune system responds by releasing histamines and other substances into the bloodstream. These chemicals cause the rashes and itching common to mild allergic reactions, as well as the life-threatening vasodilatation and tissue edema that kills people in severe, anaphylactic reactions. People who have anaphylactic reactions often, but not always, have a history of the problem, although the severity of the reaction may increase or decrease unpredictably over their lifetime.

WHEN: Allergic reactions can occur from seconds to hours after exposure, depending on the sensitivity of the person and the route by which they were exposed. The reaction may be local or systemic. A lack of previous history of sensitivity is no guarantee of immunity. Many at risk for anaphylaxis have a history of asthma. Even those aware of their allergies often do not carry proper medications.

Antigens/Allergen

Anything that can be ingested or otherwise introduced into the body has the potential to be an allergen. A significant number of reactions are called *idiopathic*, meaning no specific, known allergen is identified. Listed below are the most common allergens, but numerous others exist.

1. **Medications**: Penicillin and related antibiotics
2. **Foods:** Peanuts, wheat, nuts, milk, shellfish, eggs, and soybeans
3. **Insect stings and bites:** Bees, wasps, and ants
4. **Other:** Latex, pet dander

Signs and Symptoms

Mild allergic reactions typically involve the affected organ system with no notable changes in vital signs and no S/S of respiratory or circulatory compromise:

1. Insect stings and bites: localized itching, redness, swelling, and hives.
2. Environmental/seasonal allergies: runny nose, watery eyes, congestion, runny nose, minor wheezing
3. Minor food allergies: gastrointestinal upset, nausea, vomiting, diarrhea, facial swelling, wheezing, difficulty swallowing

Anaphylaxis is highly likely when ***any 1 of the following 3*** criteria is fulfilled following exposure to an allergen:

1. **Rapid onset of signs and symptoms with systemic skin reaction and/or mucosal tissue involvement** (e.g. generalized urticaria/hives; pruritus/itching or flushing of skin; swelling of lips, tongue, uvula, or around the eyes) **and at least 1 of the following**:

    a. **Respiratory compromise** manifested as persistent difficulty breathing, shortness of breath, and/or difficulty swallowing, stridor, hoarseness, wheezing, cough, chest tightness.

    b. **Circulatory compromise** manifested as a decrease in LOR; lightheaded/dizziness; syncope or near-syncope; weak or absent rapid radial pulses; decreased muscle tone.

Note: Criteria 1 does not require that the patient have a known history of anaphylaxis

2. <u>Two or more of the following</u> that occur rapidly after exposure to a <u>likely allergen</u> for that patient:

    a. **Systemic skin reaction and/or mucosal tissue involvement** (e.g. generalized urticaria/hives; pruritus/itching or flushing of skin; swelling of lips, tongue, uvula, or around the eyes).

    b. **Respiratory compromise** manifested as persistent difficulty breathing, shortness of breath, and/or difficulty swallowing, stridor, hoarseness, wheezing, cough, chest tightness.

    c. **Circulatory compromise** manifested as a decrease in LOR; lightheaded/dizziness; syncope or near-syncope; weak or absent rapid radial pulses; decreased muscle tone.

    d. **Persistent gastrointestinal symptoms** (e.g. painful abdominal cramps, vomiting, diarrhea, incontinence)

3. <u>Reduced blood pressure</u> after exposure to a <u>known allergen</u> for that patient:

    a. **Reduced blood pressure** manifested as a decrease in LOR; syncope or near-syncope; weak or absent radial pulses; decreased muscle tone; collapse; incontinence. When available: systolic BP of less than 90mmHg or greater than 30% decrease from the patient's baseline.

Treatment

- Remove antigens, when possible.

A: Open the mouth and assess for visible swelling of the lips, tongue, and uvula. Open and maintain the airway utilizing positioning, head tilt-chin lift, and jaw thrust in the patient with a decreased LOR. Utilize the recovery position for vomiting patients.

B: Allow the patient with difficulty breathing to assume a position of comfort. Assist respirations if necessary; provide supplemental oxygen if available.

C: Position the patient flat in the presence of S/S of shock; avoid allowing the patient to sit or stand suddenly in the presence of shock.

D: Monitor LOR as an indicator of perfusion and oxygenation status.

E: Remove any potential triggers from the environment or take actions to remove the patient from the environment where the allergen or antigen was encountered.

- Complete a secondary assessment, full set of vital signs, and patient history.
- If criteria for anaphylaxis exist, act within local or institutional protocols and assist with administration of patient's prescribed Epinephrine auto-injector in the mid-anterolateral thigh OR administration of 0.3 to 0.5 mg of Epinephrine intramuscularly to the same location. Record the time of the dose and repeat dosage in 5–15 minutes, if criteria are again met; most patients respond to 1 or 2 doses.
- If patient is responsive and can control their own airway, consider assisting the patient in taking an oral antihistamine, typically 25-50 mg Benadryl (diphenhydramine). Benadryl is NOT a substitute for epinephrine in the context of anaphylaxis.
- Reassess ABCDE, vital signs, and other complaints.

Evacuation Criteria for Allergic Reactions

1. **Rapid evacuation** if an anaphylactic reaction is suspected.
2. **Rapid evacuation** for anyone who required administration of epinephrine for S/S of anaphylaxis.
3. **Evacuate** if S/S are not alleviated by an oral antihistamine.
4. **Evacuate** if the source of allergic reaction cannot be eliminated.

Pharmacology of Epinephrine

Epinephrine (adrenalin) is a powerful drug that has multiple effects. It can save a life if given correctly to the right patient, but may also cause harm if given incorrectly or to the wrong patient. Epinephrine acts to reverse the effects of a systemic histamine release by dilating the smooth muscle of the respiratory tract and constricting peripheral blood vessels. At the same time, it has several untoward effects on the heart, including increasing its rate and oxygen demands.

Ongoing Assessment

- If possible, record a set of vitals prior to administration of epinephrine.
- Record a set of vitals soon after administration of epinephrine.
- Repeat assessment in five minutes.
- Recurrent reactions may occur up to 24 hours after initial reaction. Monitor closely. Note the availability or lack of additional doses of epinephrine.

Critical Thinking and Evacuation Criteria for Anaphylaxis

Considerable debate and misinformation surround the administration of epinephrine at the WFR/WFA level. Many states now have laws permitting the lay person to administer epinephrine. Some people regard adrenalin as the most important item in their first aid kits. Others do not even consider carrying it out of fear of litigation. The DEA is not hovering above your campsite, waiting for you to give epinephrine to yourself or your family and friends. However, administering your epinephrine to your patient (particularly if your patient is your client) without lawful protocols signed by a medical doctor can be construed as practicing medicine without a license. This is an illegal act. Similarly, it is entirely conceivable that withholding epinephrine or not having epinephrine on an outdoor trip could be considered acts of omission for which there could be serious allegations. **Understand that having a certificate that testifies to your competence in the management of anaphylaxis, including the administration of epinephrine, is no substitute for signed physician protocols that are in accordance with local laws and regulations.** To date, there are few, if any, known cases of lawsuits being brought against an individual who has administered epinephrine to the right patient in an outdoor setting.

A number of employing agencies do not have a medical director, or their medical director is not licensed in the state that the employee is working. Even so, some of these agencies expect their employees to carry and administer epinephrine if needed. This is a potential set-up for litigation. As with so many medical/legal issues, protect yourself by making informed decisions based on thorough assessments. Few lawsuits arise from positive patient outcomes.

Further mitigate your risk by considering your relationship to your potential patient and the presence of physician protocols in accordance with the law. Anaphylactic reactions evolve very rapidly, so the best time to weigh the risks and determine treatment protocols is before the trip begins.

- A person believed to have had an anaphylactic reaction should be **evacuated**, even if the reaction was successfully treated.

Evidence base for the recommendations provided in this section and additional resources:

- World Allergy Organization Guidelines for the Assessment and Management of Anaphylaxis
- Wilderness Medical Society Practice Guidelines for the Use of Epinephrine in Outdoor Education and Wilderness Settings: 2014 Update

Found at: www.aeriemedicine.com/textbook

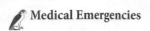

Asthma

Background

DEFINITION: *Asthma* is a transient, reversible narrowing of the lower airways. It is a disease of inflammation, spasm and secretions. The smooth muscle of the bronchioles constricts, mucus is produced in the bronchioles, and the tissue around the bronchioles swells, all impeding the ability of the patient to acquire oxygen and exhale carbon dioxide.

EPIDEMIOLOGY: The number of cases of asthma is increasing per capita globally. People may be very healthy between attacks, which might occur very infrequently. However, some individuals are highly sensitive and require daily medications to control their asthma. More often than not, persons with significant asthma have a fairly long history of it and understand its effects on them. It is crucial for you to familiarize yourself with their medicines and potential triggers before your trip so that a plan for managing an attack is in place.

Causes and Triggers of Attacks

1. Allergens: dust, pollen, pollution, smoke, molds
2. Environmental: cold, altitude
3. Anxiety
4. Exercise/exertion
5. Respiratory infections

Signs and Symptoms

1. Changes in level of responsiveness, particularly anxiety, restlessness, lethargy
2. Difficulty breathing – prolonged expiratory phase
3. Tripod position
4. Accessory muscle use
5. Wheezing or lower airway noises of constriction, primarily during exhalation
6. Decreased breath sounds (when using stethoscope)
7. Increased HR and RR
8. Skin dusky to cyanotic (depending on degree of difficulty breathing)
9. Chest pain or tightness/coughing
10. Decreased ability to talk, inability to speak in complete sentences

Treatment

A: Maintain patency (open airway).

B: Allow patient to assume a position of comfort, generally sitting upright. If patient tires, you may need to assist through rescue breathing.

C: Treat dehydration.

D: Monitor LOR as an indicator of oxygenation status.

E: Protect from extremes of temperature. Control for environmental triggers when possible.

1. Medications – Consider assisting with locating/administering rescue inhalers containing albuterol. In cases of asthmatics that experience life-threatening episodes of difficulty breathing that do not improve with rescue inhalers; administration of epinephrine may be carefully considered.
2. Hydration – Proper hydration will lessen the chances of future attacks.

Evacuation Criteria for Asthma
1. **Rapid evacuation** for any prolonged or severe attacks.
2. **Evacuate** for significantly increased frequency of inhaler use or of attacks.

Diabetic Emergencies

Background

DEFINITION: *Diabetes Mellitus ("honey urine")* is a metabolic disorder that prevents or inhibits maintenance of normal blood glucose (sugar) levels. Most often, the cause is related to an inability to utilize insulin, a hormone necessary for the entry of glucose into the cells. In some diabetics the problem is an inability of the pancreas to produce insulin.

EPIDEMIOLOGY: More than thirty million Americans, over 9% of the population, are diabetic. Nearly one in four of that population likely do not know they have the disease. It is more common in African Americans, Hispanic Americans, and Native Americans. Know your companions, students, clients, etc., and their conditions before venturing into the wilderness with them. If any are known diabetics, develop a plan and daily routine for managing blood sugar levels.

LONG-TERM CONSEQUENCES OF DIABETES: Diabetes is the seventh leading cause of death in the United States. It significantly increases the risk of stroke, heart disease, infections, blindness, hypothermia, and frostbite.

Diabetic Emergency – <u>Hypoglycemia</u> or "Insulin Shock" (hypo=low)

You are most likely to encounter patients with too much insulin relative to their blood sugar levels. These problems can manifest within minutes and require your immediate attention.

Causes of low blood sugar emergencies

1. Person **changes daily routine** (e.g., goes camping, changes diet, increases exercise)
2. Takes **normal insulin** but has a **low or inadequate caloric intake**
3. Takes **normal insulin**, eats normally, and **exercises strenuously**
4. Takes **too much insulin** for diet and exercise levels

Signs and Symptoms

1. Changes in responsiveness
2. Headache
3. "Thousand-mile stare"
4. Anxiety, restlessness, irritability
5. Sweaty, cool skin
6. Weakness (though feeling weak, these patients might fight **hard**)
7. Rapid HR and RR
8. Numbness in fingers and toes
9. Seizures
10. Unresponsiveness

Treatment

1. ABCDEs.
2. Oral sugar if they can maintain their own airway.
   - Prepare a slurry of sugar (sweetened fruit drink powder mixed rich in water).
   - Sweet candies (a soft candy bar), for them to suck on until dissolved.
   - Honey, if available, works well.
   - Follow this with more complex carbohydrates – oatmeal, rice, granola, etc.

3. If the patient has decreased LOR and cannot maintain an open airway, use the same sugar slurry and apply carefully to the gums. Glucose can be absorbed into the blood through oral mucosa, but this can take *many minutes* (upwards of 15 minutes), so wait patiently while protecting the airway. Use the recovery position to drain the airway.

4. <u>Never administer insulin</u>.

Critical Thinking and Evacuation Criteria for Diabetic Emergencies

If you are diabetic or are traveling with a diabetic, have a plan for quickly managing low blood sugar. When in doubt, a diabetic with a sudden, otherwise unexplained decrease in level responsiveness has low blood sugar.

Insulin dependent diabetics have summited Mount Everest; being diabetic and taking insulin do not preclude extended, intense backcountry activity.

1. **Evacuate** for any continuing decrease in level of responsiveness.
2. **Evacuate** if patient is unable to manage diabetes even with changes in daily routine.
3. *Consider* **evacuation** to advanced care for further evaluation if the cause of event is unclear.

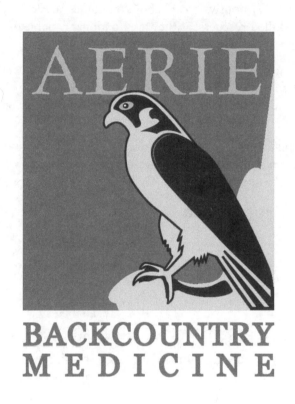

Section Six:
Environmental Emergencies

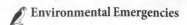

Hypothermia

Background

DEFINITION: Hypothermia is a body core temperature below 95°F (35°C). It contributes to innumerable backcountry emergencies and near-misses. Although common, the term is often misused. Most people who feel cold are not truly hypothermic. Skin cools before vital organs, causing people to feel cold, shiver, look blue, and lose fine motor skills well before their brains lose the ability to think of a way out of danger. Unfortunately, many people underestimate the significance of these early signs, choosing instead to push ahead with schedules or goals. As the brain and other vital organs cool, difficulties accelerate. Abilities to read maps, make good decisions, and perhaps most ominously, to care about outcomes, are lost. At this point, people rely on luck, vigilant companions, and skilled rescuers, as they are no longer capable of either formulating or executing their own recovery.

PREVENTION: Preventing hypothermia is easier than treating it. Stay well-fed, well-hydrated, and avoid tapping all of your energy reserves. Plan all outdoor adventures with the possibility of an unexpected night out, having the materials and/or skills for fire, shelter, water, and food. Watch your partners for early signs of hypothermia and train them to do the same for you.

NOTE: Great effort must be taken to maintain warmth and prevent hypothermia in any patient who has experienced significant trauma; this is most important in those patients who have experienced multi-system trauma or significant blood loss, whether internally or externally.

Predisposing Factors of Hypothermia

1. Dehydration
2. Exhaustion
3. Acute (short-term) malnutrition
4. Alcohol
5. Impaired shivering
6. Immobilization (due to injury or environmental factors)
7. Burns
8. Extremes of age
9. Lack of cold adaptation
10. Diabetes
11. Severe infection/sepsis
12. Spinal injuries or other central nervous system injuries

Severity

In-hospital classification of hypothermia is based on core body temperature. In the backcountry, temperatures may be difficult to obtain and are often inaccurate. Backcountry classification is determined by evaluation of the patient's LOR, movement, and shivering. The signs and symptoms listed below are highly variable.

Signs and Symptoms

- **Cold Stress** (*not hypothermic*) (Core temp. > 95°F/35°C)
    1. LOR: alert and oriented
    2. Movement: normal to slightly impaired
    3. Shivering: present
    4. HR and RR: normal to elevated

- **Mild Hypothermia** (Core temp. 90-95°F/32-35°C)
    1. LOR: alert and oriented with changes mental status (irritability, poor decision-making, apathy, lethargy begin)
    2. Movement: impaired (poor motor skills and coordination, ataxia)
    3. Shivering: active (increased shivering)
    4. HR and RR: elevated

- **Moderate Hypothermia** (Core temp. 82-90°F/28-32°C)
    1. LOR: impaired and/or decreased
    2. Movement: impaired
    3. Shivering: impaired, intermittent or absent (shivering generally ceases but may be present to 88°F/31°C)
    4. HR and RR: decreasing

- **Severe Hypothermia** (Core temp. < 82°F/< 28°C)
    1. LOR: profoundly decreased to unresponsive
    2. Movement: profoundly impaired to absent
    3. Shivering: absent
    4. HR and RR: profoundly low (assess for 1 minute before determining pulselessness/apnea)
    5. Pupils: dilated or fixed
    6. These patients may appear dead.

Treatment

- **Cold Stress**
    1. Reduce heat loss. Remove the patient from the cold and wind. Add dry clothing.
    2. Provide high-calorie food and/or drink.
    3. Encourage movement and exercise after providing calories.

- **Mild Hypothermia**
    1. Handle gently. More care must be taken to do so the colder the patient is.
    2. Direct patient to sit or lie down for at least 30 minutes before allowing other movement.
    3. Prevent further heat loss. Remove the patient from the cold and wind.
    4. Place patient in hypothermia wrap. Considerations for removing wet clothing:
        - If shelter/transport is less than 30 minutes away, place patient directly in hypothermia wrap.
        - If shelter/transport is greater than 30 minutes away, protect patient from the environment, remove wet clothing, and place patient in hypothermia wrap.
    5. Hypothermia wraps retain, but do not generate, heat. If available, apply heat to the upper trunk (anterior, lateral, and posterior upper torso) with hot water bottles or heat packs (hot rocks are not recommended). Hypothermic patients burn easily due to vasoconstriction and decreased circulation. Do not apply heat directly to the skin; reassess hourly for discoloration/redness.
    6. Body-to-body rewarming may be considered for mild hypothermia if personnel are available and it does not delay evacuation.
    7. Provide high-calorie food and/or drink.
    8. After 30 minutes of rewarming and calorie replacement an alert patient who can stand may be encouraged to exercise with low intensity.
    9. Evacuate if the patient shows no signs of improvement after 30 minutes of rewarming and calorie replacement.
    10. Remove victims from cold water in a horizontal position. They may appear mildly hypothermic (walking and talking) but remain physiologically unstable. Assess for LOR, movement, shivering, and circulatory status. Treat those immersed for 30 minutes or more as moderately hypothermic regardless of functional ability.

        NOTE: Shivering and basal metabolism are the body's most effective means of reheating. External warming measures will reduce shivering before elevation in core body temperatures occur. Support external warming with adequate caloric intake and hydration. Ensure that patients have rewarmed before you encourage significant activity.

- **Moderate Hypothermia**

  1. **Handle as gently as possible.** Avoid excessive movement of the extremities. As the heart cools, it becomes irritable. Peripheral vasoconstriction and decreased circulation result in cold acidotic blood in the extremities. Additionally, the body is hypovolemic due to cold diuresis (increased urine production). These factors and rough handling may cause cardiac arrest due to return of the cold acidotic blood to the already irritable heart.

  2. **Keep patient in a horizontal position.** Do not allow or encourage walking, standing, or movement; as much as feasible, extricate patients from water or crevasses in a horizontal position.

  3. **Prevent further heat loss.** Remove the patient from the cold and wind.

  4. Do not provide food and/or drink to the patient with a decreased LOR.

  5. Place patient in hypothermia wrap. Considerations for removing wet clothing are the same as for mild hypothermia.

     - To decrease excessive movement, consider cutting clothing away rather than manual removal.

  6. Hypothermia wraps require a heat source; they retain, but do not generate, heat. Apply heat to the upper trunk (anterior, lateral, and posterior upper torso) with hot water bottles or heat packs (hot rocks are not recommended). Take careful efforts to avoid causing burns. Heat should not be applied directly to the skin. Hypothermic patients burn easily due to vasoconstriction and decreased circulation; reassess the skin hourly for discoloration/redness.

  7. Evacuate carefully.

- **Severe Hypothermia**

  1. Follow guidelines for moderate hypothermia including gentle handling.

  2. Assess for central pulses (carotid, femoral) and respirations for 60 seconds:

     - If a pulse and/or respirations are detected: treat as moderate hypothermia.

     - If pulses or respirations are NOT detected: initiate CPR. Due to decreased metabolic demands in a hypothermic state, patients may survive prolonged CPR if transported to definitive care.

  3. Evacuate carefully.

Hypothermia Wrap

Insulate under the patient with pads to reduce conductive heat loss. Wrap the patient in a vapor barrier such as reflective blanket or plastic. Place body, including the head and neck, in insulating material. Use an outer wind proof layer to protect from convective loss via wind and rotor wash. Make an effort to remove snow and water before packaging. Place pads between patient's legs to absorb urine and feces. Neatly tuck-in all ends to avoid snow/water entering the wrap.

Critical Thinking and Evacuation Criteria for Hypothermia

1. **Evacuate** all moderate and severe hypothermia patients.

2. **Evacuate** mild hypothermia patients who do not improve with treatment.

NOTE: Do so as gently and as rapidly as feasible. Moderately and severely hypothermic patients need advanced life support and definitive medical care as soon as possible. Once in the frontcountry, hypothermic patients are not considered dead until they are *warm and dead*.

CARE FOR COLD PATIENT

SUGGESTED SUPPLIES FOR SEARCH/RESPONSE TEAMS IN COLD ENVIRONMENTS:

1 - Tarp or plastic sheet for vapour barrier outside sleeping bag

1 - Plastic or foil sheet (2 x 3 m) for vapour barrier placed inside sleeping bag

1 - Insulated ground pad

1 - Source of heat *for each team member* (e.g., chemical heating pads, or warm water in a bottle or hydration bladder), or *each team* (e.g., charcoal heater, chemical / electrical heating blanket, or military style Hypothermia Prevention and Management Kit [HPMK])

1 - Hooded sleeping bag (or equivalent)

INSTRUCTIONS FOR HYPOTHERMIA WRAP "The Burrito"

1. *Dry or damp clothing:* Leave clothing on

IF Shelter / Transport is *less than* 30 minutes away, *THEN* Wrap immediately

2. *Very wet clothing:* **IF** Shelter / Transport is *more than* 30 minutes away, *THEN* Protect patient from environment, remove wet clothing and wrap

3. *Avoid burns: follow product instructions; place thin material between heat and skin; check hourly for excess redness*

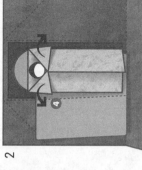

2

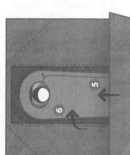

1

Tarp or Plastic

Plastic or Foil

Apply Heat

Pad

Sleeping Bag or Blanket

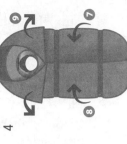

4

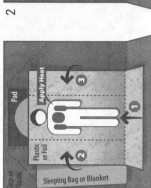

3

ASSESS COLD PATIENT

1. **From outside ring to centre: assess Consciousness, Movement, Shivering, Alertness**

2. **Assess whether normal, impaired or no function**

3. **The colder the patient is, the slower you can go, once patient is secured**

4. **Treat all traumatized cold patients with active warming to upper trunk**

5. **Avoid burns: following product guidelines for heat sources; check for excessive skin redness**

COLD STRESSED, NOT HYPOTHERMIC

1. Reduce heat loss (e.g., add dry clothing)

2. Provide high-calorie food or drink

3. Move around/ exercise to warm up

MILD HYPOTHERMIA

1. Handle gently

2. Have patient sit or lie down for at least 30 min.

3. Insulate/ vapour barrier

4. Give heat to upper trunk

5. Give high-calorie food/drink

6. Monitor for at least 30 min.

7. Evacuate if no improvement

MODERATE HYPOTHERMIA

1. Handle gently

2. Keep horizontal

3. No standing/walking

4. No drink or food

5. Insulate/ vapour barrier

6. Give heat to upper trunk

7. Volume replacement with warm intravenous fluid (40-42°C)

8. Evacuate careffully

SEVERE HYPOTHERMIA

1. Treat as Moderate Hypothermia, and

a) *IF* no obvious vital signs, *THEN* 60-second breathing / pulse check, or assess cardiac function with cardiac monitor

b) *IF* no breathing / pulse, *THEN* Start CPR

2. Evacuate carefully ASAP

(Circular diagram text:)

CONSCIOUS

IMPAIRED MOVEMENT

SHIVERING

ALERT

NOT ALERT

SHIVERING

CONSCIOUS

MOVEMENT NORMAL

CONSCIOUS

IF COLD & UNCONSCIOUS

ASSUME SEVERE HYPOTHERMIA

BICOrescue.com

Baby it's COLD OUTSIDE

Funded by the Government of Canada | Canada

Reprinted with permission.

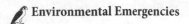

Cold Injuries

Background

INTRODUCTION

Frostnip, frostbite and cold-trenchfoot result when skin is damaged by cold. Field treatment of deep frostbite is challenging and somewhat controversial. Prevention and the recognition of early signs and symptoms of these conditions are essential.

PHYSIOLOGY

- Blood flow to the skin can vary from 25 ml/minute to 7,500 ml/minute.
- Blood easily bypasses hands, feet, nose and ears by shunting the blood through arterio-venous *anastomoses*.
- **Direct contact** with cold causes vasoconstriction (e.g., touching a cold ice axe).
- **Indirect cold** causes vasoconstriction (e.g., a cold head makes cold hands).
- Dehydration reduces the ability to circulate blood.
- Adaptation to cold is primarily through increased **cold-induced vasodilatation** (anastomoses periodically open, allowing blood to reach extremities).

PREVENTION

- Bring proper equipment and extra hats, gloves, and over-mitts.
- Maintain a warm core during activity by adding, subtracting or changing clothing layers.
- Cover all skin to prevent contact vasoconstriction. Use liner gloves.
- Maintain hydration and nutrition.
- Use hand-warmers in gloves and boots.
- Check on your partners! Check fingers, toes, face and ears regularly.
- Wind-milling arms is very effective at forcing blood back into hands.
- Avoid contact with water, metal, or gas – flash-freezing risk.
- Avoid constrictive clothing (tight leggings, boots, etc.).
- Be especially careful if you have a history of previous cold injury.
- Do not ignore numb toes/finger etc.

Specific Cold Injuries

1. Frostnip

Definition: Superficial, temporary near-freezing of tissues, especially the nose, cheeks, fingers and toes.

Signs and Symptoms

1. Pain, often tingling, possible numbness
2. Pallor – white, waxy color

Treatment

1. Remove any wet clothing and replace with warm, dry clothes.
2. Apply heat. Place cold hands in groin or armpits, put feet on partner's abdomen, use warm hands to cover an area with possible cold injuries.
3. Prevent further exposure, as this area may be more susceptible to future cold injury.

2. Frostbite

Definition: Freezing injury of tissues, with destruction of cells. Similar to burns, frostbite can range from damaging the epidermis and dermis only (superficial) to freezing the full thickness of an extremity. These wounds are at high risk of infection.

Signs and Symptoms

1. **Superficial**:
   - Before re-warming: Pale, numb skin. Tissue remains pliable.
   - After rewarming: Early-forming clear blisters extending to tips of digits.
2. **Full-thickness**:
   - Before rewarming: Skin is hard, white, waxy and numb, sometimes burgundy.
   - After rewarming: Late-forming (or absent) dark, isolated blisters which, if on a completely frozen extremity, do not extend to the tips of the digits.

Treatment

1. **Superficial Frostbite – Field Rewarming**
   - **Water Bath Technique**: A warm water bath between 100-102^{0}F (38-39^{0}C) should be maintained for 30 minutes until circulation is restored. (Expect this to be PAINFUL!) Keep in mind the practical challenges involved in rewarming by this method: frozen tissue, small pot of water, limited quantities of water, limited fuel supplies, difficulties maintaining let alone simply measuring water temperatures. You must also avoid contact of the injury with the container. Which is why skin-to-skin rewarming (see below) may be the most practical option.
   - **Body-to-Body Contact (without rubbing!)**: Often the most realistic treatment in a backcountry environment. Place frostbitten hands against the skin in armpits or groin. Negotiate a bribe to place bare, frostbitten feet on a partner's bare abdomen.
   - **Protect the Injury** from pressure, friction, further trauma, and especially re-freezing. Wrap the fingers and toes as you would a burn.
   - **Consider ibuprofen** for pain and swelling.

2. **Full-Thickness Frostbite**
   - **Leave frozen if there is the possibility of re-freezing.** Field re-warming of full-thickness frostbite should not be considered unless evacuation will take many hours or days. How long is not absolute and will depend on patient condition, distance to definitive care, and immediate resources.
   - **Dress and insulate the injury**: Wrap the injury with gauze sponges between fingers or toes and loosely surrounding the injury. Insulate the area with non-cotton material and cover with a windproof layer.
   - **Protect/splint the injury** from further injury, cold and pressure.
   - **DO NOT** warm with the **radiant heat** of a fire or field stove as this will likely burn the tissue. **Do not break blisters.** If spontaneous thawing occurs **do not allow to re-freeze**. **Do not rub.**

NOTE: There are continuing developments and recommendations for the field treatment of frostbite. Most of the recent recommendations, however, involve advanced therapies that must be mitigated within the first 12-24 hours after the tissue has frozen. This is well outside of the practical evacuation window that we will operate within in the field. In these cases, field-rewarming may be our best option. We must understand that if we are withholding rewarming until after evacuation, frostbitten tissue will often passively thaw and refreeze during evacuation. This cycle further harms previously damaged tissue. To complicate matters, this thawing-but-still-frozen tissue will continue drawing heat away from a body that is most likely already struggling to maintain its own heat balance.

Evacuation Criteria for Frostbite

All frostbite injuries, including those rewarmed in the field, need clinical evaluation.
If less than 2 hours from care, **evacuate immediately** for rewarming, assessment, and pain management.

3. Trenchfoot

Definition: Trenchfoot is a non-freezing injury (usually of the feet) caused by prolonged, often cold, wetness. This results in intense vasoconstriction, decreased circulation and skin cell death.

Prevention: Similar to frostbite prevention. Allow feet to dry every night. Reserve one pair of dry socks for sleeping. Dry wet socks on bare torso overnight. Do not wear wet socks for long periods of time. Foot powder can be helpful.

Signs and Symptoms

- Symptoms rarely develop in less than 4 days.
- Feet appear cold, swollen, and waxy with burgundy to blue splotches.
- Later stages, feet become red and hot with blisters.

Treatment

- Remove wet socks and allow feet to dry out. Dry boots if possible and put on dry socks.
- Protect from freezing.
- Consider ibuprofen for pain and swelling.

Evacuation Criteria for Trenchfoot
Evacuate for S/S of infection.

High Altitude Illnesses

Background

CAUSES: The suite of illnesses seen at elevation are due to a combination of decreasing oxygen levels and decreasing atmospheric pressures. All people are susceptible to altitude illness, but to varying and largely unpredictable degrees.

WHERE: Most cases of altitude illness are seen at elevations above 8,000 feet (2,400 meters); although, it is observed as low as 5,000 feet (1,500 meters).

PHYSIOLOGY: Faced with decreasing oxygen levels, the body compensates within minutes by increasing its respiratory rate and depth. While necessary and highly adaptive, this increases blood pH, requiring increased urination to buffer the change. While also necessary, this dehydrates a body that is already challenged to maintain hydration. Over the course of numerous days, the body begins to acclimatize in other ways including, increasing red blood cell production and increasing its ability to efficiently carry and use oxygen. Acclimatization does not preclude altitude illness, and is not related to a person's fitness level.

PREVENTION

- Maintain hydration despite a lack of thirst.
- Maintain nutrition despite a lack of appetite.
- Climb high and sleep low.
- Ascend gradually; 2,000 feet/day above 8,000 feet (600 meters/day above 2,400 meters).
- Pay attention to past history of altitude illness.
- Maintain a high index of suspicion for any changes in behavior or ability to walk. Altitude illness can mimic and sometimes exacerbate dehydration, hypoglycemia, head injuries, respiratory infections, exhaustion, and even overdoses.
- Consider prophylactic use of Diamox® (acetazolamide).

Acute Mountain Sickness (AMS)

AMS is the most common discomfort experienced at elevation. Its symptoms most likely result from swelling in and around the base of the brain, and symptoms result from reduced oxygen concentrations and atmospheric pressure. Severity is dependent upon (1) rate of ascent, (2) absolute altitude reached, and (3) individual susceptibility (related to physiological and anatomical factors). The onset is often gradual, and it is easy to confuse with other conditions. Maintain a high index of suspicion when at altitude.

Signs and Symptoms

Mild AMS feels much like a hangover

1. Headache –worse in early morning, related to nocturnal periodic breathing
2. Dizziness, nausea
3. Fatigue
4. Disturbed sleep, loss of appetite

Severe AMS is a further progression of the above symptoms, plus:

1. Altered LOR/ataxia
2. Rales (fluid sounds in lungs)
3. Cyanosis, shortness of breath at rest
4. Poor overall impression (lassitude → unresponsiveness → death)

   NOTE: Severe AMS is **life-threatening** and can progress to other forms of altitude illness.

High Altitude Cerebral Edema (HACE)

Definition: A progression of the cerebral symptoms and altered LOR in persons with AMS.
Physiology: Evidence suggests that minor brain swelling occurs in the majority of newcomers to altitude, even as low as 5,000 feet (1,500 meters). Susceptible individuals have increased cerebral blood flow and increased intracranial pressure (ICP). Neurologic compromise results from increasing ICP.

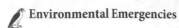

Signs and Symptoms
1. Any of those associated with AMS
2. Altered LOR
3. Ataxia
4. Nausea/vomiting
5. Vision disturbances (tunnel vision, blindness, etc.) and/or hallucinations
6. Unresponsiveness → death

High Altitude Pulmonary Edema (HAPE)

Definition: A progression of AMS in which fluid accumulates in the alveoli and membranes of the lungs. Pulmonary function decreases as fluid accumulates. Sometimes misdiagnosed as pneumonia. HAPE is the most common cause of non-traumatic death at elevation.

Physiology: Pulmonary blood flow dynamics change at the capillary level in susceptible people. Higher than normal pressures in pulmonary arteries cause leakage of fluid into alveoli, as well as an accumulation of fluid in the walls of the alveoli. Respiration is inhibited either by decreased area for gas exchange or by increased distance oxygen must travel.

Signs and Symptoms
1. Any of those associated with AMS or HACE
2. Shortness of breath (first, with activity; later, at rest)
3. Weakness
4. Rales (sound of fluid in lungs)
5. Coughing fits, progressively more severe. Progressively more productive and frothy
6. Bloody or pink frothy sputum
7. Cyanosis
8. Unresponsiveness → death

Treatment for Altitude Illnesses
1. Hydration, rest, and nutrition for mild AMS.
2. **Descent for Severe AMS, HAPE, or HACE.** Descent is the only definitive treatment. If possible, go down 1,500-3,000 feet or more (450 to 900 meters or more). One cannot descend too quickly.
3. Supplemental oxygen, if available.
4. Pressure-breathing (pursed lips during exhalation).
5. Gamow® bag for hyperbaric oxygenation, if available.
6. Medications available by prescription: acetazolamide, dexamethasone, albuterol, nifedipine, sildenafil.

(No one treatment replaces the need for adequate acclimatization before symptoms appear, or immediate descent once afflicted.)

Critical Thinking

Hypoxia from high elevations puts a stress on the body that can mimic, hide, or exacerbate other medical problems. A general rule of thumb is that problems at altitude, particularly those associated with changes in levels of responsiveness, should be considered altitude illness and treated with descent until proven otherwise. One general plan for treatment of suspected but unconfirmed altitude illness is to "Treat the Fearsome Fives":

1. Food (Hypoglycemia)Weak
2. Fluids (Dehydration)
3. Fahrenheit (Hypothermia and Hyperthermia)
4. Fatigue (Exercise Exhaustion)
5. Feet (Altitude – Hypoxia)

Evacuation Criteria for Altitude Illness

Evacuate/descend for signs and symptoms of severe AMS, HAPE or HACE.

Lightning

Background

PREVALENCE: Lightning strikes occur in an instant with tremendous force and energy. About 25 million strikes hit the ground each year in the United States, accounting for approximately 50 deaths per year. Lightning is unpredictable and occurs in any outdoor setting. Strike survivors, who account for about 90% of those struck, can have life-long deficits from the accident. Although lightning can (and does) strike anywhere at any time, it tends to occur more frequently in the summer months. Statistically, lightning will strike most often during the afternoon and early evening. Most people injured are not struck directly; instead they are near an object that has been struck. Chances of being injured can be minimized by practicing lightning safety techniques.

A fully-enclosed building offers the most protection from lightning. Vehicles with a hard-top frame provide the next best option. These should be utilized if closely available. Be aware many people are struck by lightning while moving towards safer areas.

PREVENTION:

1. **Recognize Danger**

   - Learn to read the weather and *pay attention to it*. It is easier and safer to avoid high-risk areas than bail off a ridge in the middle of a storm. Research the area you plan to travel and know the weather patterns there.

   - Be aware of the landscape around you. Look for signs of previous strikes in the area.

   - Watch for warning signs such as hair standing on end, buzzing sounds, skin tingling, and/or a faint glow from objects at night.

   - **Flash/Bang:** Count the number of seconds it takes to hear thunder following a lightning flash. *Note*: Sound generally travels one mile (1.6 km) every five seconds (faster at sea level, slower at higher elevation).

   - **5-Second Rule:** If the flash/bang is 5 seconds or less, <u>immediately</u> get to location of safety.

   - **30-30 Rule:** If the flash/bang is 30 seconds or less, go to a safer place and stay away from locations of danger for at least 30 minutes after the last flash/bang.

2. **Locations of Danger**

   - Descend from summits, ridge tops, and other exposed locations, and squat down in the lightning position. (It is more effective to change your geographic position rather than your physical posture).

   - Move away from water. This includes indoor plumbing.

   - Move away from tall objects like trees and rock outcroppings. Move a distance at least twice the height of the object.

   - Move away from cave entrances, overhangs and rock walls, especially when wet.

   - Avoid large open meadows.

   - Stay away from any device that has wires connected to electricity or a wall socket.

3. **Locations of Safety**

   - Spread everyone in a group 20 to 40 feet (6 to 12 meters) apart.

   - Seek shelter in growths of small trees of uniform height.

   - Assume the lightning position by sitting/squatting on an insulating pad or other non-conductive object. Keep your feet together, cover your ears and tuck your head.

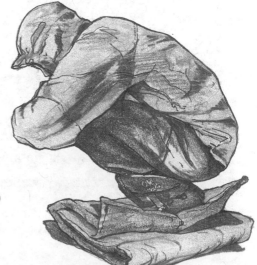

Lightning Position

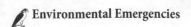

Signs and Symptoms

Mortality is most commonly attributed to one of two causes:

1. Cardiac arrest and subsequent respiratory arrest
   - Heart stops immediately after strike due to electrical disruption
   - Respiratory system arrests due to lack of oxygen
   - Heart spontaneously resumes beating
   - Respiratory center does not spontaneously resume
   - Second cardiac arrest results from cardiac hypoxia
2. Neurological injuries – Brain hemorrhage or other CNS damage due to electrical current

Injuries to Organ Systems

1. **Cardiac**: Cessation of cardiac rhythm and/or damage to heart tissue
2. **Respiratory**: Inhibition of respiratory drive
3. **Nervous System**
   - Loss of responsiveness
   - Confusion/amnesia
   - Seizures
   - Transient or permanent paralysis
4. **Skin**: Feather burns and/or true thermal burns; temporary extremity cyanosis from vascular smooth muscle spasm
5. **Musculoskeletal**: Dislocations, fractures, or other blunt force trauma; muscle spasms, muscle necrosis
6. **Ears**: Ruptured eardrum from sound waves, hearing loss and ringing
7. **Eyes**: Loss of vision, cataract formation

Treatment

Two Unique Features of Lightning Strike Emergencies:

1. Efficacy of CPR – CPR may prevent a fatal hypoxia due to the initial cardiac arrest of a lightning strike.
2. Triage – Due to the above feature, treat the "dead" first in multiple-patient incidents involving lightning strikes. Do not triage out pulseless and apneic victims of lightning unless they have been down for prolonged periods or have signs incompatible with life.

Other Injuries

1. On each patient, treat injuries as found based on severity as you would for any other traumatic injury. Examine for entry and exit wounds from the strike. Inspect for burns resulting from jewelry, zippers or melted clothing.
2. Suspect spinal injuries – lightning's explosive forces may result in high-impact blunt-force trauma.
3. Suspect hypothermia - electrical disruption of CNS may obstruct thermoregulatory mechanisms.
4. Treat burns as any other burn.

Evacuation Criteria for Lightning Strike Patients

1. **Evacuate** all lightning strike patients.

Drowning

Background

PREVALENCE:

Globally, approximately 372,000 people die from drowning each year, with an average of 4,000 occurring annually within the United States. These numbers exclude deaths that occur during floods or other natural disasters. For every incident of fatal drowning, there are 4 or more incidents of nonfatal drowning. Nonfatal drowning injuries may result in brain damage with long-term disabilities such as memory problems, learning disabilities, and permanent loss of basic functioning (permanent vegetative state). Drowning is one of the 10 leading causes of death for people aged 1-24 years in every region of the world. It is the second leading cause of death in 1 to 4 year olds. A common drowning scenario is a male patient who cannot swim, did not intend to enter deep water, is not wearing a personal flotation device (PFD), and is intoxicated.

DEFINITIONS:

Drowning: The process of experiencing respiratory impairment due to submersion or immersion in liquid. Only three outcomes are possible: (1) mortality; death (2) morbidity; survival with medical complications (3) no morbidity; survival without medical complications. More simply, drowning can be either fatal or not.

Terms and categorizations that should not be used with drowning: near, secondary, delayed, wet, dry, active, passive, saltwater, or freshwater.

Mammalian Dive Reflex: A debatable body response when cold water contacts receptors in the back of the nose, slowing the metabolism and vital organs and shunting blood to the brain.

CAUSES OF DEATH AND INJURY:

Death from drowning is caused by lack of oxygen to the brain. Brain death often occurs after a sequence of struggle in the water, breath holding and unconsciousness, with very little water actually absorbed into the lungs. Contributing factors to mortality and morbidity include pulmonary edema from a loss of surfactant in the lungs and pneumonia.

Immersion Syndrome: Sudden cardiac arrest immediately after submersion in very cold water.

Circum-rescue Collapse: A phenomenon occurring immediately before, during, or shortly after rescue from cold water. Symptoms range from fainting to cardiac arrest due to an inability to maintain heart function, blood pressure, and body temperature, especially when horizontal positioning is not maintained.

PREVENTION:

- Evaluate the risks and benefits of students, clients, and/or companions swimming in the backcountry.
- In alpine lakes, cold water may cause respiratory problems in people with pre-existing respiratory conditions like asthma. This is true even for experienced swimmers more accustomed to warm ponds and pools. Use extreme caution when crossing any streams deeper than your knees, particularly with packs on. Consider crossing in groups to provide support.
- Wear a properly-fitted personal flotation device (PFD) and helmet when operating in or near water.
- If alone in the water, assume HELP position (heat-escape-lessening posture). A personal flotation device (PFD) is necessary.
- If with a group in the water, face inward and huddle with arms interlocked. A PFD is necessary.

Outcome Determinants of Submersion

Outcomes of submersion incidents are generally based on two factors:

1. **Submersion Time**: The shorter the better. The vast majority of patients submerged for greater than 15 minutes will not survive.
2. **Water Temperature**: Cold water survival times are better (upwards of an hour), though survival rates decline rapidly after 15 minutes.

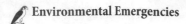

Treatment

Don't Become a Victim: Hello, Reach, Throw, Row, Go, Helo (helicopter)

1. Remove patient from the water. Maintain horizontal positioning for those immersed in cold water. Providing spinal motion restriction (SMR) should never distract from the immediate priorities of airway management and rescue breathing and should not endanger rescuers or unnecessarily delay extrication from the water. Provide initial SMR for those involved in an unknown or specific mechanism of injury that may result in spinal injury, such as diving. Further maintenance of SMR should be provided to unreliable patients (altered or decreased LOR) or those with S/S of a spinal injury.

2. Do not attempt compressions in the water.

3. Begin with 5 rescue breaths on all apneic (not breathing) patients. Respiratory arrest usually precedes cardiac arrest, so immediate ventilation may allow for spontaneous circulatory resumption. If it does not delay extrication or put rescuers at risk, ventilate the apneic drowning patient (referred to as *In Water Resuscitation*, or *IWR*) patient during extrication from the water.

4. If CPR is begun (after extrication), ensure that it includes effective ventilations.

5. Provide supplemental oxygen when available.

6. For prolonged immersion in cold water (greater than ½ hour) treat for hypothermia, even if the patient appears stable. Extricate the patient in a horizontal position and treat as gently as is practical. Hypowrap the patient and apply heat to the upper torso following recommendations listed in the hypothermia section. If the patient appears lifeless, prioritize airway management, ventilations, and compressions when indicated while simultaneously providing rewarming measures.

Evacuation Criteria for Drowning

1. **Evacuate** unresponsive patients or those who lose consciousness in the water.
2. **Evacuate** patients with a decreased or altered level of responsiveness.
3. **Evacuate** patients requiring rescue breathing.
4. **Evacuate** patients who develop signs of respiratory distress up to 24 hours after the event.
5. **Evacuate** patients who exhibit a persistent cough after the incident.
6. **Evacuate** patients who exhibit frothy sputum or foamy material from their airway.
7. **Evacuate** patients who exhibit signs of low blood pressure (weak or absent distal pulses).
8. **Evacuate** patients with pre-existing respiratory diseases.
9. **Evacuate** patients with pre-existing heart problems or persistent rapid heart rates post event.

Heat Emergencies

Background

PREVALENCE: Heat emergencies are extremely common in outdoor settings.

CAUSES: They are caused by imbalances of water, electrolytes, and heat in the body. These factors do not necessarily occur concurrently.

PREVENTION: In any of the heat-related conditions, acclimatization reduces the incidence and severity of injury. Acclimatization requires daily activity in a hot environment for 1½ to 2 weeks, and confers four primary advantages: (1) a lower sweating threshold, (2) elevated sweating rates, (3) decreased electrolyte loss in sweat, and (4) more effective cooling through elevated skin blood flow.

PHYSIOLOGY: Heat loss is accomplished through radiation (#1 in temperate climates), evaporation (#1 during exercise or in hot climates), conduction, and convection. Ambient humidity decreases the effectiveness of evaporative cooling.

Heat Cramps (Exercise-Associated Muscle Cramps)

Definition: Muscle pain and spasm (usually legs and abdomen) following water and electrolyte loss.

Signs and Symptoms

1. Severe pain and cramping in muscles and abdomen, associated primarily with exercise
2. Rapid pulse
3. LOR usually alert and oriented
4. Normal to slightly increased body temperature

Treatment

1. Move patient to a cool environment. Rest for 1-2 hours. Massaging and stretching may help.
2. Provide 1-2 liters of water with electrolytes or supplemental salty foods as tolerated by patient.
3. Monitor vitals – if body temperature is elevated and/or persistent with significant decrease in LOR, consider heat exhaustion and/or heat stroke.

Heat Syncope

Definition: A sudden, transient loss of consciousness (or near loss of consciousness) and postural tone (control of body position) that resolves promptly with supine positioning, rest, removal from heat, and hydration.

Signs and Symptoms

1. A brief, complete or partial loss of consciousness during upright positioning
2. Rapid pulse
3. Pale, sweaty
4. LOR after event quickly returns to alert and oriented with supine positioning
5. Normal to slightly increased body temperature

Treatment

1. Lay patient flat.
2. Move patient to a cool environment. Rest for 1-2 hours.
3. Provide 1-2 liters of water with electrolytes or supplemental salty foods as tolerated by patient.
4. Monitor vitals – if body temperature is elevated and/or persistent with significant change in LOR, consider heat exhaustion and/or heat stroke.

Heat Exhaustion

Definition: Patient loses water and electrolytes (usually through exercise) and becomes dehydrated. This is a form of hypovolemic shock.

Signs and Symptoms

1. Skin is pale and clammy with profuse perspiration; or slightly flushed
2. Headache, dizziness, fatigue, weakness, syncope (fainting), irritability
3. Nausea/vomiting, loss of appetite
4. HR = rapid, weak
5. RR = shallow and rapid
6. Body temperature = slightly elevated above normal (< 104°F, or 40°C)

Treatment

1. Move to a cool, shaded environment. Rest and cool for 12-24 hours.

2. Lay the patient flat.
3. *Slowly* rehydrate the patient, starting with about 200 ml/hr, as patient can tolerate.
4. Facilitate evaporative cooling by sponging with cool water and fanning the patient.
5. Record vitals. If LOR is significantly altered, treat for heat stroke.

Exertional Heat Stroke

Definition: A true life-threatening emergency in which the body's cooling mechanism fails. Often, overexertion with low fluid replacement in a hot, humid environment brings on this condition. Other patients may have pre-existing medical conditions or an acute medical event, such as a stroke, that leaves them unable to care for themselves in the heat.

Signs and Symptoms

1. Decreased or altered LOR: confusion, disorientation, agitation, hallucinations, etc.
2. May be no warning before sudden collapse and unresponsiveness
3. Headache, dizziness
4. Seizures
5. Skin warm or hot to touch; may be flushed and dry (classic heat stroke) or wet (exertional heat stroke)
6. Body temperature >104°F (40°C); rectal temperature being most reliable
7. Rapid HR and RR

Treatment

1. ABCDEs - maintain an open airway and provide continuous monitoring during cooling measures.
2. Immediately remove from heat and initiate rapid cooling of the patient.
   - Most effective: Remove clothing and immerse patient's torso and extremities in cold water.
   - Less effective: Remove clothing, sponge with cool water, and fan patient
   - Least effective: Apply cold packs to groin, armpits, head and neck.
3. Do not administer fever reducers (Tylenol®, aspirin).
4. Continue to monitor while evacuating. The person is at risk for other complications.

Exercise-Associated Hyponatremia

Definition: Lower than normal blood sodium concentration occurring during or up to 24 hours after prolonged physical activity.

Cause: Typically caused by excessive fluid consumption during continuous endurance exercise lasting greater than 4 hours. EAH is complex and its diagnosis can be difficult in the out-of-hospital environment. Primary prevention strategies involve avoidance of fluid consumption in excess of sweat loss.

Signs and Symptoms of critical EAH (may present hours after the activity ends)

1. Changes in LOR: confusion, disorientation, agitation, hallucinations, unresponsiveness
2. Seizures
3. Respiratory distress due to pulmonary edema (fluid shift into the lungs)
4. Headache, dizziness, blurred vision
5. Ataxia, lack of coordination
6. Fatigue, weakness
7. Nausea/vomiting
8. Clear, copious urine output (decreased or absent urine output is also possible)
9. Peripheral edema of hands, feet, face (acute weight gain in some instances)
10. Normal body temperature (possibly slightly elevated)

Treatment

1. Rest, cool, and remove from heat if applicable.
2. Rule out dehydration or other conditions with similar S/S before proceeding with additional treatment.
3. For patients who can maintain their own airway: consider providing high salt food or a hypertonic solution such as 3-4 bouillon cubes in 125 ml of water.

Evacuation Criteria for Heat Emergencies

1. **Rapidly evacuate** patients with suspected heat stroke.
2. **Evacuate** patients unable to tolerate oral fluids for 24 hours or more.
3. **Evacuate** patients with a change in LOR.

Carbon Monoxide (CO) Poisoning

Background

DEFINITION: Colorless, odorless, and tasteless, carbon monoxide is an insidious gas produced by the combustion of organic fuels. No matter how efficient your camp stove may be, it produces CO and should not be used indoors.

PHYSIOLOGY: CO affects the central nervous system (CNS) by impairing the circulatory system. Hemoglobin (the oxygen-carrying protein in red blood cells) has over 200 times the affinity for CO than it does for oxygen. Thus, oxygen must compete with CO in the circulatory system. A healthy person at sea level can take over four hours to exhale CO. The recovery time more than doubles at high altitude.

Signs and Symptoms

CO poisoning may mimic or exacerbate other problems, especially acute mountain sickness (AMS). Maintain a high index of suspicion for both AMS or CO poisoning based on the setting and other findings.

1. Dizziness
2. Confusion
3. Headache
4. Lethargy to coma
5. Respiratory arrest
6. Skin may be pale to cherry red, though this is often a late sign. Cyanosis usually occurs first.

Treatment

1. Protect yourself. Rescuers can be overwhelmed in minutes by CO.
2. Remove patient(s) from confined space and assure adequate ventilation.
3. Ensure ABCDEs.
4. If apneic or breathing is otherwise inadequate, provide rescue breaths.
5. Administer high-flow oxygen, if available. Otherwise assure patient is breathing fresh air.

Critical Thinking and Evacuation Criteria for CO Poisoning

Very experienced mountaineers and outdoors people have died from CO poisoning. Suspect it with any unexplained mental status change in an enclosed setting (e.g., tent, snow cave) or when multiple people are altered in a confined space. Do your absolute best to never cook in your tent or snowcave.

Evacuate patients with suspected CO poisoning or change in LOR.

Stings, Bites, and Rubs

1. Hymenoptera

Bees, wasps, hornets, and ants.

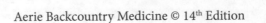

Treatment of Insect Stings

1. Scene safety (many stinging insects are territorial).
2. Remove the stinger quickly, if applicable. Use care, if possible, to not squeeze the venom sac if still attached to the stinger. Otherwise, there is no preferred method for removing a stinger; just get it out.
3. ABCDEs - Assess for signs and symptoms of anaphylaxis and assist appropriately.
4. Consider application of neutralizing agents (meat tenderizer or papaya powder), acids like citrus (e.g., a slice of lemon) for wasps/ hornets; bases/ drawing agents (e.g., baking soda) for bees; and local cold compresses for pain.
5. Consider antihistamines to minimize local signs and symptoms.

2. Arachnida

Spiders and scorpions. All spiders are venomous. People are notoriously bad at identifying the culprit, and spiders get blamed for far more unexplained wounds than they deserve.

Spider bites in the U.S. are uncommon, and when they do occur, are usually harmless because most bites are unable to penetrate human skin, and most toxins do not react with mammals.

Two types of spiders whose bites have the potential to cause harm: Black Widow and Brown Recluse.

- **Black Widow:**
  - Very common.
  - Only females envenomate. Bite is painful.
  - The majority of bites cause only local skin irritation, but bites that result in true envenomation can be of clinical significance.
  - The neurotoxin causes painful, sustained muscle spasms that begin several hours after the bite.
  - Spasms can be so severe that they mimic the pain of a ruptured appendix or kidney stones.

- **Brown Recluse:**
  - Found in North and South America.
  - Both male and female envenomate.
  - Most bites result in mild, localized skin irritation.
  - The venom causes vasospasm and can result in skin necrosis that can extend far beyond the wound site.
  - Necrotic lesions are concerning because they carry high risk for infection and require aggressive wound care.

Treatment of Spider Bites

1. Stay calm. Keep patient calm.
2. Clean the wound.
3. Treat anaphylaxis as a life-threatening problem.
4. Antivenin exists for black widow bites, but generally only helps in severe cases.
5. Once a patient starts to exhibit muscle spasms from a black widow, even if localized, they should be evaluated in a hospital for symptom control.

Evacuation Criteria for Bites and Stings

Most unexplained, small wounds in the United States that get ascribed to spider bites are probably infected wounds having nothing to do with a spider. Therefore, good wound management is essential. Regardless, **evacuate** for pain, tissue damage, signs of systemic effects, infection and/or for further evaluation.

Aerie Backcountry Medicine © 14th Edition

3. Ticks

Background: Ticks require mammalian blood as part of their life cycle. They possess highly-developed mouth parts for attaching to and acquiring blood from hosts. Ticks are transmitters (vectors) capable of spreading disease. They are vectors for Rocky Mountain spotted fever, Colorado tick fever, Lyme disease, and other diseases including typhus, viral encephalitis, etc.

Prevention: Check yourself and others daily when in tick country. Remove ticks carefully. Consider using Permethrin or other insecticides on clothing.

Tick Removal

1. Specialized tick tweezers are helpful (narrow and pointed).
2. Grasp tick as close to skin as possible. Pull gently and steadily. It does not matter what direction you pull the tick out.
3. Treat the wound for infection and monitor for up to two weeks.

Lyme Disease

Ticks transmit many diseases; amongst these, Lyme disease deserves particular mentioning.

- The most common tickborne infection in the United States and Europe.
- Caused by *Borrelia burgdorferi*.
- Most commonly carried by the deer tick, *Ixodes scapularis* and *Ixodes pacificus*.
- It can be transmitted in the early stages of the tick's life, when they are no bigger than the tip of a pen.

Signs and Symptoms

1. Redness around site
2. Red rash, referred to as "Erythema Migrans" (literally, migrating rash) that may or may not be itchy, that often spreads from the site of the tick attachment (usually appears within a month).
3. Malaise
4. Low grade fever
5. Muscle/joint pain and swelling
6. Other symptoms, including cardiac and neurologic, occur over months to years if not treated.

> ### Evacuation Criteria
> **Evacuate** for any s/s of tickborne illness after exposure to ticks, particularly with a known or suspected bloodfeeding.

4. Mammal Bites

Treatment

Mammal bites are often nasty things: puncture wounds contaminated with bacteria suited to thrive in the harsh conditions of an animal's mouth.

1. Clean these wound thoroughly.
2. Flush with copious amounts of water and iodine.
   - Repeat.
3. Look for more wounds and don't ignore "minor" scratches.

Rabies

A fatal viral infection that debilitates the central nervous system (CNS). Primary hosts in the US include wild animals such as bats, raccoons, skunks, and foxes. Worldwide, dogs account for 99% of human deaths from rabies. In the US, deaths are rare, with most fatalities occurring in people who fail to seek medical attention, typically because they were unaware of an exposure.

Signs and Symptoms

1. Insomina
2. Anxiety
3. Headache
4. Confusion
5. Fever
6. Abdominal pain
7. Change in behavior
8. Seizures

NOTE: Once signs and symptoms appear (typically two to ten days, but, rarely, can manifest after more than a year), death usually follows within days and all treatment attempts will be unsuccessful.

Treatment

- Irrigate site thoroughly, preferably with a virucidal agent (povidone-iodine or chlorine dioxide) or soap and water, and evacuate to a medical facility capable of administering prompt postexposure prophylaxis (PEP).

> ### Evacuation Criteria for Mammal Bites
> **Evacuate** all mammal bites that break the skin.

5. Hantavirus Pulmonary Syndrome (HPS)

Background

- Caused by the *Sin Nombre* virus carried by some mice and rats (deer mouse; cotton rat; rice rat; white-footed mouse). These are not typically the animals that live in most residences other than cabins and structures surrounded by woodlands.
- Caused by the inhalation of mouse urine, saliva, or feces contaminated with the hantavirus.
- Since 1993, >700 cases have been diagnosed.
- Mortality is approximately 36%.

> #### High-Risk Areas
>
> › **Large deer mice populations**
> › **Living spaces infested with mice**
> › **Visible deer mouse droppings**
> › **Opening/cleaning unused buildings or structures**
> › **Cleaning areas with little use (e.g., sheds, attics)**

Prevention: Use caution when in high-risk areas. Wear surgical face masks and gloves, and clean suspected contaminated areas with 10% bleach solution.

Signs and Symptoms

Universal Early:	Occasional Early:	Universal Late:
• Fatigue • Muscle Aches (especially large-muscles and back)	• Headache • Dizziness • Chills • Nausea	• Coughing • Severe Shortness of Breath

> ### Evacuation Criteria
> **Evacuate** patients with suspected HPS and provide comfort.

6. West Nile Virus

Background

- Transmitted by female mosquitoes, typically of the *Culex* species.
- 36 of 200 mosquito species in the U.S. carry the virus.
- As of 2019, mosquitoes caused human infections in 49 states.
- 150 asymptomatic cases per one severe case.
- 1 in 5 people infected develop a fever and other symptoms.

Prevention: DEET or other repellents.

Signs and Symptoms

1. Usually occur within 2-15 days
2. Sudden fever, malaise
3. Nausea/vomiting
4. Occasional rash

Evacuation Criteria

Evacuate patients with suspected West Nile Virus and provide comfort.

7. Snake Bites

Prevention

- Watch for snakes in late afternoon and along river banks during evenings and dry seasons. Become familiar with the habits of the snakes in your area.
- If a snake is encountered, back away slowly. Snakes can strike well over half their body length.
- Wear appropriate boots in snake country.
- **Do not** attempt to chase, catch, or otherwise handle snakes.
- **Do not** handle dead snakes or detached heads as they can have intact bite reflexes.

Crotalinae: Pitvipers (rattlesnakes, water moccasins, copperheads)

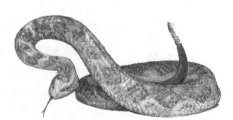

- 99% of envenomations in the U.S. are from pitvipers.
- 50% occur when purposefully handling the snake.
- 90% in U.S. occur in warmer summer months when snakes are more active.
- Of the 7,000-8,000 venomous snake bites that occur annually in the US, approximately 5 are fatal.

Signs and Symptoms of Crotalid Envenomation

1. Venoms are complex and reactions are variable.
2. Pain, swelling, blisters and/or continuous bleeding/oozing at the site.
3. Some report a metallic taste, numbness, and tingling.
4. Severe envenomation may progress to shock, respiratory arrest, unresponsiveness, and death.

Treatment

"There is nothing that can be done in the field to significantly alter the outcome of a serious snakebite, and field first aid should not delay rapid transfer to a facility capable of safely administering antivenom." – WMS Practice Guidelines for the Treatment of Pitviper Envenomations in the US and Canada

1. Scene safety. Get the patient and other people away from snake.
2. Remove or cut jewelry or other constrictive items from affected extremity – swelling will occur.

3. **"The 3 Rs"**
   - **Rest:** Keep the patient still as you complete your assessment and implement your evacuation plan.
   - **Reassure:** Calm the patient. Implement psychological first aid.
   - **Rapid evacuation:** Seek medical attention as quickly as possible. Carefully implement rapid evacuation to an appropriate facility; this may require self-evacuation.
4. Quickly clean/irrigate the wound with soap and water and apply a sterile dressing.
5. Using a permanent marker, circle the bite site and write the time the bite occurred on the patient. Approximately every 30 minutes mark the leading edge of redness and swelling and write the time on the patient. Document other S/S.
6. Splinting may have minimal positive effect and must not interfere with circulation as swelling occurs. Loosely splint or immobilize the extremity in a position of function at the level of the heart, when possible.
7. Anaphylaxis from snake bites is rare. If the criteria for anaphylaxis occur administer epinephrine as indicated.
8. **DO NOT** apply any form of a pressure dressing to pitviper bites.

Elapids: Coral Snakes

- Occur naturally in the southern US, Central, and South America.
- Venom is primarily neurotoxic.
- Envenomation occurs from a chewing bite.

Signs and Symptoms of Elapid Envenomation

1. Chewing bite.
2. Pain, swelling, and/or blisters at the site.
3. Neurological signs and symptoms such as numbness, tingling, eyelid heaviness.
4. Severe envenomation may progress to shock, respiratory arrest, unresponsiveness, and death.

Treatment

1. Scene safety. Get patient and other people away from snake.
2. Remove or cut jewelry or other constrictive items from affected extremity.
3. **"The 3 Rs"** –see above.
4. Follow additional care as listed for Crotalinae.
5. Although recommended for elapid envenomations outside of North and South America, application of a pressure-immobilization bandage for coral snakes of the Americas remains an unproven therapy.

NOTE: For all crotalid and elapid bites; **DO NOT** cut the site, **DO NOT** attempt to suck out the venom, **DO NOT** apply a tourniquet, **DO NOT** apply ice or immerse in water, **DO NOT** apply electricity, **DO NOT** administer NSAIDS such as Aspirin, Ibuprofen, Naproxen, **DO NOT** administer or apply alcohol, **DO NOT** attempt to bring the snake with you either dead or alive.

Evacuation Criteria for Snake Bites

Rapid evacuation to a facility capable of antivenom administration for all snakebites. This may not be the closest hospital or clinic.

Evidence base for the recommendations provided in this section and additional resources:

- Wilderness Medical Society Practice Guidelines for the Treatment of Pitviper Envenomations in the United States and Canada

Found at: www.aeriemedicine.com/textbook

8. Rubs: Allergic Contact Dermatitis

Toxicodendrons: Poison Ivy, Poison Oak, Poison Sumac

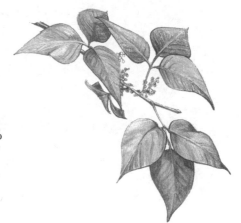

- Members of the family *Anacardiaceae*, the cashew family.
- Identification is the key to prevention. Sayings such as "leaves of three, let it be" are practically useless, as many harmless plants have three leaves while members of the cashew family are leafless in their dormant state but nevertheless still contain urushiol in their stems. It is better to take the time to learn the plants of areas you will be visiting.
- Urushiol is the allergenic resin in stalks and leaves – about 50% of U.S. population is sensitive.
- Urushiol binds to the skin in a short period. None will wash off after 60 minutes without specific cleansers. Blisters developing later do not contain urushiol.
- Resin remains active on, and may be spread by contact with, animal hair, clothing, and tools.

Prevention

1. Learn to identify the plants.
2. Wash yourself immediately after exposure.
3. Use protective clothing.

Signs and Symptoms

1. Onset typically occurs 24-48 hours after initial exposure
2. Localized redness, swelling, itching, and burning
3. Formation of blisters
4. Possible systemic reactions (anaphylaxis)

Treatment

1. Wash skin as soon as possible with cold water and soap or specific cleansers (e.g., Technu® Oak-N-Ivy Cleanser® and Dr. West's Ivy Detox Cleanser®).
   - Cold water alone is somewhat effective because urushiol is moderately water-soluble.
2. Cool compresses decrease pain.
3. Oral antihistamines such as diphenhydramine (Benadryl®) and levocetirizine (Xyzal®) might help.
4. Topical creams might be mildly effective at reducing weeping lesions and itching. Hydrocortisone cream applied at the earliest stages has been shown to be mildly effective.
5. Topical applications of cornstarch, baking soda, oatmeal or aloe vera juice help relieve itch.

Evacuation Criteria

1. **Evacuate** for persistent reactions.
2. **Evacuate** for severe local signs and symptoms (especially marked blistering and/or swelling).
3. **Evacuate** for signs and symptoms of infection.

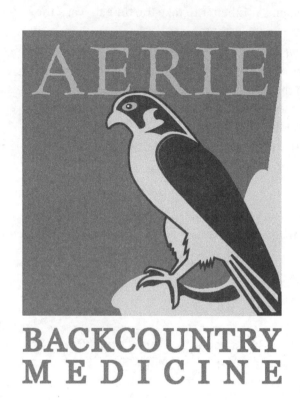

Section Seven:
Decision Making

Backcountry Decision Making

Background

GOALS: Due to the absence of black and white answers to important questions, backcountry emergencies pose unique challenges. Rescuer needs, patient needs, and group needs are of absolute priority at every step of the process, as is gathering and sorting information for proper decision-making. As an outdoor leader with responsibility for friends, family, clients, students, or even as an independent traveler with some medical knowledge, others may look to you for guidance and order during a potentially chaotic situation. This role requires an efficient system for gathering information, formulating a plan that addresses the needs of those involved, and delegating responsibility to others. While each event or situation will be unique, the system used for decision-making in the backcountry can be essentially universal.

DEVELOPING A PLAN: Just as developing a plan is important for patient assessment, it is also critical when managing the scene and evacuation. Backcountry situations usually require a more comprehensive evaluation of the resources available, the personnel available, the patient's condition, the number of patients, the location and environmental conditions, and the condition of the remainder of the group. Considering each of these components is essential to ensuring proper patient care and group safety. However, it need not be overwhelming and can, in fact, be relatively straightforward. A plan is a guideline to keep everybody safe. If the plan needs to change, change it, but only for a good reason. Developing contingency plans is especially helpful in the ever-changing backcountry environment.

PREVENTION: Developing a strategy for possible evacuation before entering the backcountry is the best way to mitigate many of the complications that are bound to arise during an emergency situation. This includes forethought on communications (e.g., radio, cellular or satellite telephones, satellite messenger device, personal locator beacon, etc.), terrain hazards and evacuation routes, skills among your group, and the other possible resources available to you.

DETAILS: Careful planning takes time. Recognize this and your stress will be reduced greatly. STOP and think. The operational principle in developing an effective plan is prioritization; taking the extra few minutes to organize your thoughts and consider the options will allow you to prioritize well.

Elements of Decision Making

1. **Scene Survey**
   - Scene Safety
   - Number of Patients – Is everyone accounted for?

2. **Patient Assessment**
   - Primary Survey
   - Triage if there are multiple patients – Sort by injury/patient priority
   - Secondary Survey

3. **Patient Needs**
   - Injury Severity
   - Injury Management
   - Ambulatory Status

4. **Situational Variables**
   - Group status: nutrition, hydration, rest, number
   - Location: distance, terrain, time of day, and season
   - Weather: worsening/clearing, wind, precipitation
   - Resources available: splint/litter materials, personnel, camping gear, communications gear, first aid kits, etc.

5. **Developing a Plan**
   - Should you stay or should you go?
   - How/when will you go?
   - Do you require assistance?

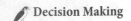

Evacuation Criteria

"He who neglects what is done for what ought to be done, sooner effects his ruin than his preservation." --Machiavelli, The Prince

Background

Nobody likes to be told to go home. Most of us invest a considerable amount of time and effort getting outdoors, and an evacuation means leaving our goals behind. If you are working in the backcountry, there may be financial incentive to stay and leaving may require absence from gainful employment. While some injuries and illnesses absolutely require evacuation, most are not that straightforward. As always, use your best judgment and any protocols of your company or organization (if they apply). The detailed evacuation criteria included in the chapters of this manual will serve as good guidelines; so can the following summary of conditions leading to the decision to evacuate.

Evacuate Patients Exhibiting these Signs and Symptoms:

1. ABCDE problems
- Anaphylaxis; current or resolved with epinephrine
- Severe asthma attack; current or resolved
- Persistent shortness of breath from any cause
- Unexplained, persistent chest pain
- Signs and symptoms of shock

2. Neurologic Deficits, Altered Mental Status
- Loss of consciousness/changes in level of responsiveness that is related to a medical/traumatic condition or cannot be explained
- Changes in vision or speech
- Asymmetric smile/facial droop
- One-sided weakness and/or arm drift
- Unexplained weakness
- Seizures
- Progressing S/S of mild head injury
- S/S of severe head injury

3. Musculoskeletal trauma
- Known or suspected fracture
- Sprain or strain that impairs the patient's ability to move on their own >24 hours
- Persistent inability to bear weight
- Dislocations (resolved or not)

4. Fever, nausea & vomiting, diarrhea
- Signs of sepsis with suspected source of infection
- Fever, N/V, diarrhea persisting for >24 hours
- Particularly with signs of dehydration/hypovolemia
- Abdominal pain lasting >8 hours (immediate evacuation if sudden onset of severe pain)

5. Spinal Injuries
- Significant trauma to body (MOI) *and*
- Unreliable patient
  - a. Anything other than A&Ox4 (unaware of person, place, time, or event)
  - b. Distracting injuries; long bone fractures
  - c. Impairment from alcohol, drugs, emotions
- Signs and symptoms of spinal injury
  - a. Spinal pain or tenderness
  - b. Decrease or change in sensation or movement of extremities
    - Numbness/tingling
    - Inability to feel pain or light touch
    - Weakness or paralysis
  - c. Signs of trauma to the spine

6. General
- Many causes for evacuation do not fit into tidy categories, but are nonetheless justified.
- Consider evacuating patients for:
  - a. **Psychological crisis & behavioral emergencies** are challenging to identify and quantify, and should be managed by a mental health professional. Suicidal intent or ideation expressed by the patient requires evacuation. The stable but otherwise listless, unhappy person may be prone to injury and unreliable in an emergency.
  - b. **Mechanism of injury** although an unreliable predictor of injury, MOIs such as high falls, significant force, etc. should be considered in your decision making. Note the young healthy patient's ability to compensate, potentially masking S/S of significant trauma.

Triage and Multiple Casualty Incidents

Background

DEFINITION: Triage is the act of sorting multiple patients by injury priority, based on the resources available and other situational variables. Done during times of high stress, triage is both calculated and imprecise. Coordinating many rescuers, allocating limited resources and making decisions to achieve the greatest good for the greatest number are difficult tasks in themselves. Adding the intense emotion that a multiple-casualty incident potentially generates results in an extremely stressful situation for all involved.

DETAILS: All situations are different, and all triage decisions are dependent on the situation. Circumstances can change quickly, and the decision-making process needs to be flexible enough to accommodate this. Triage is implemented based on the Incident Command System (ICS), in which a central leader delegates tasks to officers in charge of certain duties (Triage Officer, Logistics Officer, etc.). Communication during these stressful events is most efficient when using a chain of command.

Patient Triage

Patients are generally sorted by priority in a system that assigns a color based on injury severity.

Treat patients in the following order:

1. **Red** – Most critically injured: Altered LOR, problems with ABCDEs, life-threatening wounds
2. **Yellow** – Less critically injured. Limb-threatening wounds
3. **Green** – Non-life- or limb-threatening wounds, "walking wounded"
4. **Black** – Patients who are pulseless and apneic or have injuries that preclude survival

   NOTE: This order of treatment priority is subject to change (e.g., lightning strike patients assigned 'black' may receive treatment first).

Steps in Performing Triage:

1. **Designate the following:**
   - **Incident Commander** (IC): Person in charge of overall incident; responsible for decision-making, assignment of other roles, maintaining organization and communication. Should perform little or no patient care. May be located off site.
   - **Triage Officer**: Should be the most experienced care provider – if experience is equal, choose the person with the best organization, communication, and leadership skills.
   - **Safety Officer**: Should be in charge of overall scene safety, including rescuers' hydration, nutrition, rest, psychological status, and environmental hazards.

2. **Simple Triage and Transportation Phase** – Triage Officer conducts a 30-60 second assessment of respirations, perfusion, and mental status on all patients and assigns them a color. After triage assessment, move patients to treatment sectors based on color assigned:
   - **Immediate Care Sector** – Treat Red then Yellow – Those who will be helped the most by immediate intervention.
   - **Delayed Care Sector** – Treat Green - Those who will live no matter what is done.
   - **Non-salvageable Sector** – Treat Black - Those who are likely to die no matter what is done.

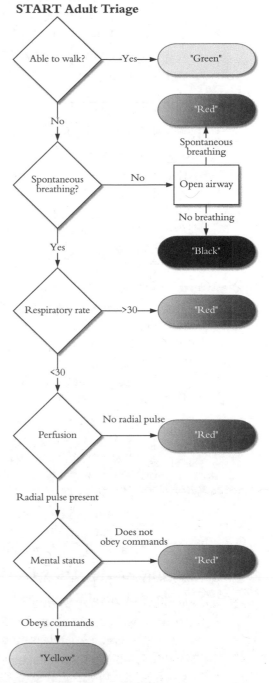

START Adult Triage

Able to walk? —Yes→ "Green"

No

Spontaneous breathing? —No→ Open airway

Spontaneous breathing → "Red"

No breathing

Yes

"Black"

Respiratory rate —>30→ "Red"

<30

Perfusion — No radial pulse → "Red"

Radial pulse present

Mental status — Does not obey commands → "Red"

Obeys commands

"Yellow"

3. **Patient Care Phase** – Provide care based on priority. Triage Officer should refrain from providing care other than directing resources, recording information about all patients, and reporting information to the Incident Commander.

4. **Re-evaluation Phase** – Triage Officer performs secondary triage of all viable casualties, communicates to IC. Triage Officer and caregivers continually re-evaluate patient condition and priority.

Communications

1. The Incident Commander needs information about the status of all activities.
   - Patient care, transportation, resource and equipment needs and availability, rescuer status, etc.
   - All officers need to report at regular intervals.
2. Communication flows two ways in the Incident Command System – top-down and bottom-up.
3. Keep radio traffic concise and less than 30 seconds per transmission.
4. Written records facilitate organization. SOAP notes are essential.

Stress Management

Potential Stressors Encountered During Emergencies and EMS Operations

Stress injuries may result from exposure to a single event or multiple exposures over time.

1. **Patients, Families, and Bystanders**
   - Suffering, pain, injury, disease or death
   - "Senselessness" of pain and suffering
   - Rude, demanding, unreasonable, or threatening people
2. **Interventions**
   - Feeling of failure and guilt
   - Patient demise in spite of care-givers' successes
   - Feeling of not being able to do enough
3. **Coworkers**
   - Apparent dishonesty and selfishness
   - Thinking that you were more a part of the problem than the solution
   - Miscommunication with team members
4. **Environmental**
   - Dangers: driving, weather, patients, weapons, toxic chemicals
   - Workplace: hours, lights and noises, sharing quarters with others, lack of privacy
   - Health: poor diet/nutrition, disrupted/poor sleep health
5. **Families**
   - Irregular hours
   - Emotional involvement that leaves others feeling confused or diminished
   - Separate worlds – lack of understanding
   - If several family members work in EMS, danger of excessive preoccupation with work

Managing Acute Stress During an Emergency

1. **Physiological Responses**
   - Sympathetic Nervous System releases stress hormones causing an increase in BP, HR, RR, dilated pupils, and glucose release into the blood.
   - Beneficial, to an extent, in an emergency; potentially harmful if left unmanaged long term.

2. **Managing a Stress Response**
   - Utilize performance-enhancing breathing, positive self talk, visualization, and a focus word or phrase to help control your physiologic response.
   - File it, but understand that if not addressed such events may be stored in memory and may lead to development of stress injuries.
   - Focus on immediate attainable goals.
   - Performing under stress takes practice, maintain realistic expectations for yourself.

3. **Strategies for Interacting with the Patient and Family**
- Utilize the concepts of Psychological First Aid.
  - Promote a sense of safety.
  - Promote calming.
  - Promote a sense of self- and collective-efficacy.
  - Promote connectedness.
  - Promote hope.
- Be respectful, clear and concise, and honest in your communications.
- Anticipate potentially dysfunctional situations/behavior.
- Don't expect to be unaffected.
- Know the rules regarding resuscitation and Do Not Resuscitate (DNR) orders.

Signs of Stress Reaction After an Emergency

1. **Physical**
- Disrupted sleep patterns; insomnia or sleeping too much, fatigue, exhaustion
- Increased or decreased eating
- Increased drinking or drug use; numbing, "self-medicating"
- Hyperarousal, hypervigilance, exaggerated stress response

2. **Psychological**
- Intrusive memories, thoughts, images, emotions
- Avoidance of similar stimuli, activities, events
- Depression, anxiety, hopelessness, guilt, lack of interest, tearfulness
- Anger, impatience, irritability
- Confusion, memory lapses, inability to concentrate, dissociation
- Withdrawal from family, friends, sex, activities and interests, isolation

After an Emergency: Stress Management Techniques and Resources

1. **Stress Management Techniques**
- **Care of Your Mind:** Commit to good self-care, reach out to trusted family and friends, journal, practice mindfulness, cultivate healthy interest and activities, build and trust in your own resilience, speak with a mental health professional.
- **Care of Your Body:** Eat regular nutritious meals; avoid or limit alcohol, caffeine, and sugar consumption; exercise regularly; establish and maintain healthy sleep habits.

2. **Resources**
- National Suicide Prevention Lifeline: www.samhsa.gov, 1-800-273-8255
- www.codegreencampaign.org
- www.responderalliance.com
- www.revivingresponders.com
- EMS, Safe Call Now: www.safecallnow.org, 1-206-459-3020

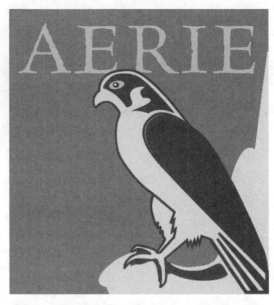

Section Eight:
Utilities

Water Purification and Filtration

Background

Many individuals never treat their water and are apparently none the worse for it. However, unfortunately much of the world's freshwater is contaminated with harmful pathogens, and contaminated water kills and incapacitates *countless* numbers of people. Treating water is prudent, and to do this effectively you need to consider the most likely contaminants in that water and understand the most effective means of eliminating them.

Methods of Purification

I. Heat

- Boiling is reliable.
- Simply bringing water to a boil provides adequate disinfection for most water. However, harmful chemicals and pesticides from farmland run-off are not usually mitigated with boiling water.
- Remove all particulate debris from water before boiling.
- Boil water for 1 minute at elevations below 6,000 feet (1,800 meters) and for 3 minutes above 3,000 feet (900 meters).
- It typically takes 1 kg (2.2 lb) of wood to boil 1 liter of water.

II. Chemical Treatment

- Halogens: Iodine and Chlorine are usually used in tablet, liquid, crystalline, or resin forms.
- Effectiveness depends on:
  a. Concentration once applied to water
  b. Contact time
  c. Water temperature
  d. Amount of organic impurities in the water
- **To increase the palatability and effectiveness of halogens:**
  a. After required contact time, add ascorbic acid (vitamin C) to change iodine and chlorine into iodide and chloride, both of which are tasteless.
  b. For turbid water, allow water to settle (1-2 hours) and decant by slowly pouring water into another container as to avoid particulates that have settled at the bottom. Consider adding alum (1 pinch of pickling salts per gallon) as a coagulant and flocculent, and decant water a second time.

  #### 1. Iodine and Chlorine
  - Simple and largely effective against giardia, bacteria and most viruses. They are unreliable against cryptosporidium.
  - An open bottle of iodine loses 30% effectiveness over 4-5 days.
  - Iodine has an effect on the thyroid gland of a developing fetus. Don't use if you're pregnant.
  - Inconclusive studies on the long-term effect of iodine use. It is recommended that iodine not be used extensively for more than 2 months.
  - Chemical activity slows in colder water.
  - Halogens bind with impurities, causing them to disinfect much more slowly or to require significantly higher dosages to attain disinfection.

  #### 2. Chlorine Dioxide
  - ClO_2 is a very effective virucide, and is capable of eliminating most bacteria and protozoans from water.
  - It is available in granules, tablets, and as a liquid.

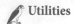

III. Filtration

- Effectively filtering microorganisms from water depends on the pore size of your filter. Be familiar with your equipment. Most filters are unreliable at removing viruses.

- Although your filter may say that it will remove most common pathogens, keep in mind that microorganisms can bend and squish under pressure and may sneak through a single pore. For this reason, if you have doubts about the contents of your water, pre-treat it with iodine or chlorine and then filter it.

- Some filters on the market incorporate an iodine resin into the unit, combining filtration and chemical treatment. The iodine is held in a matrix that water contacts as it is filtered, and such a small amount of iodine is released that it is virtually tasteless.

- Ceramic filters manufactured by Katadyn© do contain small enough pores to remove most, if not all, pathogens, including viruses. They tend to be expensive and heavy, though, and may crack if dropped or frozen. They may work well for prolonged base-camps.

IV. Ultraviolet (UV) light

- Ultraviolet water disinfection uses short wave light rays to deactivate the DNA of bacteria, viruses and other pathogens. In particular, it interrupts their ability to reproduce and multiply and therefore their ability to make us sick.

- Advantages are that it is safe with no exposure to chemicals, no changes in taste, odor or pH of water and simple to use.

- Particulate matter in the water can shield the pathogen from UV exposure and therefore not disinfect the water. For maximum efficacy, use with a filtration system to remove particulates.

- Another disadvantage is the dependence on a battery-operated device in the backcountry.

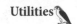

First Aid Kits
Background

The exact contents of a first aid kit will depend on the specifics of the outing including location, activity, duration, number of people and their levels of training, among other factors. Often, multiple kits are present for longer outings. Coordination of these decreases weight and increases function.

First aid kits must be versatile and lightweight and must contain items you know how to use. Having a well-stocked kit is good, but having the skills to use it is better. Think creatively and improvise what you can. This means thinking of multiple uses for your gear at home, before you embark. Never learn how to use something under duress. Go through your kits frequently to restock and relearn their contents. **Consult a physician** regarding the use of any medication you plan to administer.

Bleeding Control	Infection and Blister Control	Medications (see Medications)	Splint/ Tape	Accessories/ Utilities
4" ACE® Bandage	Irrigation syringe	Pain	SAM® Splint.	2 pairs of non-latex surgical gloves
4x4s (gauze pads)	Moleskin or adhesive-knit bandage	Allergies	2" athletic tape (duct tape may suffice)	Light source (headlamp or flashlight)
Rolls of 3" or 4" roll gauze	Second Skin for minor burns or blisters	Infection	Cravats (triangular bandages)	Pencil
4" Self-adhesive wrap	Compeed® or Blistoban® for blisters	Burns		SOAP Notes
Large absorbent dressing (e.g., 5x9" gauze pad)	Tincture of Benzoin swabs or other tacky skin prep	Upset Stomach		Cotton applicators
		Diarrhea		Scissors or trauma shears
Tourniquet	Alcohol prep pads	Sun		
		Teeth		Tweezers
Hemostatic agent	Spyroflex® or other bio-occlusive dressings			Safety pins
	Band-Aids®			Write-in-the-Rain® paper
	Steri-strips®			CPR face shield or Pocket-Mask
	Povidine iodine for 1% iodine solutions			Thermometer
	Telfa® or other non-adherent dressing			Duct Tape
				Glucose Tablets or Paste

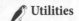

Medications

Depending on trip details, you may choose to carry medications in your kit. You should be familiar with everything you carry and have some form of literature to reference when using it. Keep medications in their original containers, if possible, to avoid problems with customs or other officials. The CDC recommends that travelers consult the embassy of the country they will be visiting, and that they be exceedingly cautious about traveling with narcotics and other controlled substances. Continually refresh your kit with new medications, as it is easy to let them expire and not notice until you need them most. Although it is prudent practice to safeguard medications, many remain effective despite extremes of temperature, humidity, and light.

It is possible to obtain prescriptions for medications from physicians before you leave for extended trips or to other countries. Consult with a travel medicine physician or travel clinic before going abroad. If you are taking medications for client use, you must have medical oversight/protocols for all medications, no matter how benign they are. The following are general suggestions. There may be serious side effects and contraindications not listed. **Always consult with a physician for indications and complications of any medicine you carry.**

Medications are listed with generic names first followed by common trade names in parentheses. If there are differences in use for a given category, some of the uses are listed last.

Note: Medications purchased abroad may not meet the same standards as those purchased within the US.

Non-prescription Pain Meds

Acetaminophen (Tylenol®):..............................Pain, Fever
Aspirin (ASA, Bayer®, Ecotrin®): ....Pain, Fever
Non-Steroidal Anti-Inflammatory Drugs (NSAIDs)
Ibuprofen (Advil®, Motrin®, Nuprin®):........Pain, Swelling, Fever
Naproxin (Aleve®):..................................... Pain, Swelling

Prescription Pain Meds

Codeine
Hydrocodone (Vicodin®)
Other narcotic analgesics (pain relievers)

Non-prescription Antihistamines

Diphenhydramine (Benadryl®, Diphen®): ...... Allergic Reactions

Prescription Meds for Anaphylaxis/Asthma

Epinephrine (EpiPen®):........... Vasoconstriction/Bronchodilator
Inhalers- Albuterol. (Ventolin®):.......................... Bronchodilator

Non-prescription Antacids

Famotidine (Pepcid®)
Calcium Carbonate (Rolaids®, Tums®)

Non-prescription Gastro-Intestinal (GI) Meds

Bismuth subsalicylate (Pepto-Bismol®):.................Anti-diarrheal
Loperamide (Imodium®, Kaopectate®): ....Anti-diarrheal
Senna (Dosalax®): .... Stool Softener

Prescription Gastro-Intestinal (GI) Meds

Diphenoxylate/atropine (Lomotil®):.......................Anti-diarrheal

Prescription and Non-prescription Nasal Decongestant

Pseudoephedrine (Afrin®, Sudafed®)

Prescription Giardia Med

Metronidazole (Flagyl®)

Prescription Antibiotics

Broad spectrum antibiotics
Azithromycin (Zithromax®)
Specific antibiotics
Azithromycin (Zithromax®):..........................Traveler's Diarrhea
Ciprofloxacin (Cipro®): ....Traveler's Diarrhea
Cephalexin (Keflex®): .... UTI, Bites, Wounds

Prescriptions for High Altitude

Acetazolamide (Diamox®) ....Prevention/treatment of AMS
HAPE, HACE
Albuterol..Treatment for HAPE
Dexamethasone .... Treatment for HACE
Nifedipine.. Treatment for HACE
Sildenafil ....Treatment for HAPE

Prescription and Non-prescription Topical Ointments

Aloe gel: ....Superficial Burns
Hydrocortisone (Cortizone®):..................................Hives
Anti-biotic cream/ointment (Neosporin® Polysporin®).....Minor cuts and scrapes
Glucose
Sunscreen
Lip ointment
Oil of cloves:... Dental pain
Lidocaine: ....Abrasions, gum pain
Tetracaine Ophthalmic: ....Eye abrasions

Travel Medication

Appropriate vaccinations and immunizations information at:
www.travel.state.gov
www.cdc.gov
www.who.int/en
www.osac.gov

Traveling with controlled substances:
www.incb.org/incb/en/travellers/country-regulations.html

Traveling with medicines:
wwwnc.cdc.gov/travel/page/travel-abroad-with-medicine

Preparedness and Survival Considerations

Background

Backcountry travel involves risk and includes the potential to transition into an emergency scenario. Beyond injury or illness, miscalculations of route, terrain, weather, speed of travel, and/or other situational variables may lead to a wilderness emergency. It is worth noting that many worst-case scenarios were not single cataclysmic events, but a series of small mistakes neither acknowledged nor acted upon.

As with so many things in wilderness medicine, prevention is paramount. Conscious decision-making with an ongoing awareness of your surroundings is fundamental. Decision-making includes communication of physical needs, limits, and abilities and should include an awareness of terrain, weather, and potential hazards specific to your activity. The ability to accurately navigate cannot be over emphasized; dependency on a single technology to do so should be avoided.

In addition to the medical skills needed to manage a patient in an extended care situation, many wilderness emergencies require the ability to provide for the survival needs of oneself, party, and patient. A planned and practiced means of providing shelter and warmth, hydration, nutrition, and an ability to communicate to potential rescuers should be considered a minimum. Prior practice and preparation will enhance your ability to function under the stress of a wilderness emergency.

Prior preparation includes communication of your itinerary to a dependable third party as well as having an emergency response plan. Do not be afraid to discuss worst-case scenarios with your group. Instead, plan for them.

Physiological Requirements and Survival Priorities

1. Psychological: ability to manage stress response and maintain cognitive function
2. Oxygenation: adequate oxygen exchange and delivery
3. Thermoregulation: ability to maintain core body temperature
4. Hydration: adequate water intake
5. Nutrition: adequate caloric intake
6. Rest, Recovery, and Elimination: adequate sleep, rest, and hygiene
7. Acclimatization: to altitude and other environmental variables when relevant
8. Protection: from environmental extremes, sun, wind, precipitation, insects, animals, etc.
9. Injury and Illness: ability to provide first aid for oneself and others
10. Navigation: ability to accurately determine location and follow a planned route
11. Signaling and Communication: ability to communicate distress and location to a third party

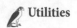

Survival Kit Contents
"The Backcountry Bomb Shelter"

Similar to a first aid kit, the contents of a survival kit should reflect the environment, activity, and skill level of it[s] user. It must be versatile and lightweight, simple and easily utilized under stress. You should be fluent with the gear you are depending on. Use it, practice with it, and review it frequently. Tailor it to your needs and couple i[t] with existing gear you already carry.

Protection	Navigation/ Weather	Communication/ Illumination	Utilities/ Additional
*Equipment specific to the environment and activity	*Compass	*Headlamp with extra bulb and batteries	*Knife or multi-tool
*Clothing utilizing base layer, mid layer, and outer layer including waterproof shell	*Topographical map of area	*Pea-less whistle	Packable handsaw
Extra base layers and socks	Global Positioning System (GPS)	Chemical glow stick	*50-100 feet cordage
Gloves/mittens, stocking cap/ balaclava	Watch	Emergency light (e.g. blinking bike light or beacon)	Extra batteries
Bandanna	Altimeter	Signal panel	*Duct tape
Sunglasses/goggles		Write-in-the-Rain® notepad	Freezer bags
Sunscreen and lip balm		Pencil/Sharpie®	Safety pins
Bug spray and permethrin treated clothing as appropriate		Cell phone- with ability to recharge	Sewing needles
Bear spray as appropriate		Personal Locator Beacon or Satellite Messaging device	Floss
Chemical hand/toe warmers			Picture frame wire
*First aid kit			Zip ties
			Toilet paper
			Flat magnifying glass
			Water proof container

Shelter	Water	Fire	Food
*Quality space blanket or bivy	*Water bottle	*Strike anywhere matches with striker in waterproof container	*Quick energy foods- consider honey or favorite candy
Tarp space blanket or alternative tarp/ground cloth	*Collapsible water container	*Butane Lighter	Energy bars to your liking
Alternatives:	*Purification tablets	*Cotton balls saturated in Vaseline in waterproof container	Other light weight emergency food items
Bivy sack	Lightweight filter or UV system	Ferrocerium fire rod with striker	Consider a source of caffeine
2 Large heavy duty trash bags, preferably orange leaf bags	Metal container for boiling water	Candle	
	Length of tubing for water collection		

* Signifies items considered essential or items whose light weight and value allow them to be easily carried.

Helicopter Landing Zone

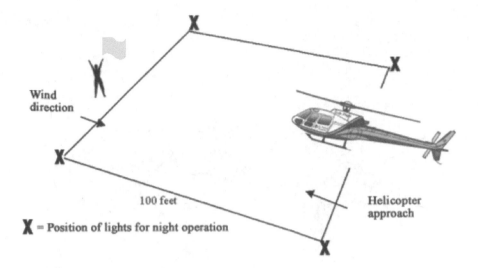

Wind direction

100 feet

X = Position of lights for night operation

Helicopter approach

Preparing a Helicopter Landing Zone (LZ):

1. Designate a Landing Zone Officer (LZO) to communicate with the helicopter crew.

2. LZ must be at least 100' x 100', flat, firm, and free of all obstacles. It should ideally be 200-500 feet from the patient care area to avoid rotor wash blowing dust, debris, snow, or materials.

3. LZO must be visible and identifiable from the air (i.e., wearing an orange vest and using a flashlight).

4. LZO will report wind speed, direction, and any hazards to the pilot via radio, when possible.
   - Helicopters approach and depart the LZ facing into the wind.
   - Telephone and electrical wires and metal cables are very difficult to see from the air, especially at night. Communicate the presence of any in the area.
   - Flagging or similar material may provide a wind gauge visible by the pilot from the air.

5. Illuminate LZ with non-flammable lights. Assure no lights are pointed upwards toward the helicopter.

6. As the helicopter approaches, the LZO will stand with back to the wind and hands raised above head.

7. The LZO needs to move out of rotor wash area but maintain eye contact with pilot.

8. Pilot may opt for a different LZ after flying over the area.

9. The LZO should maintain radio silence during approach and take off unless communicating emergency information to the pilot.

10. Assure that no one approaches the helicopter unless directed by the crew. Only approach the helicopter if and when directed by the crew, approach and leave the helicopter as specifically directed by the crew, staying in sight of the pilot.
    - Wear eye and ear protection.
    - Avoid the front and back of the helicopter. Do not go near the tail rotor of the helicopter.
    - Only approach from down slope if on uneven terrain. Do not approach from up hill.

11. Follow instructions from the crew when assisting with loading.
    - Secure any loose items.
    - Keep objects below shoulder level.
    - Depart as a group.

12. As helicopter departs, LZO will keep area clear and report any hazards to pilot.

Abdominal and Thoracic Anatomy

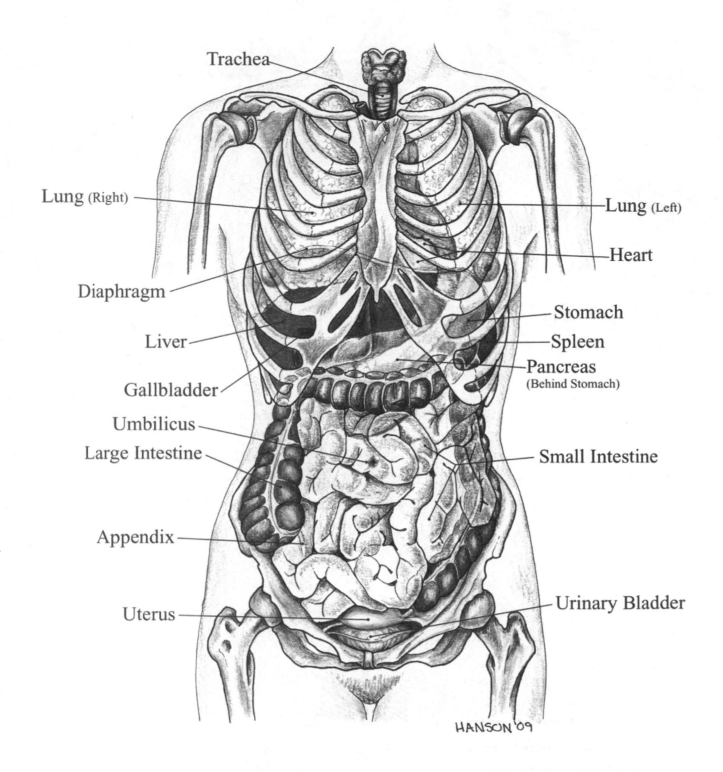

Trachea

Lung (Right)

Lung (Left)

Heart

Diaphragm

Stomach

Liver

Spleen

Pancreas
(Behind Stomach)

Gallbladder

Umbilicus

Large Intestine

Small Intestine

Appendix

Uterus

Urinary Bladder

HANSON '09

Skeletal Structure Anatomy

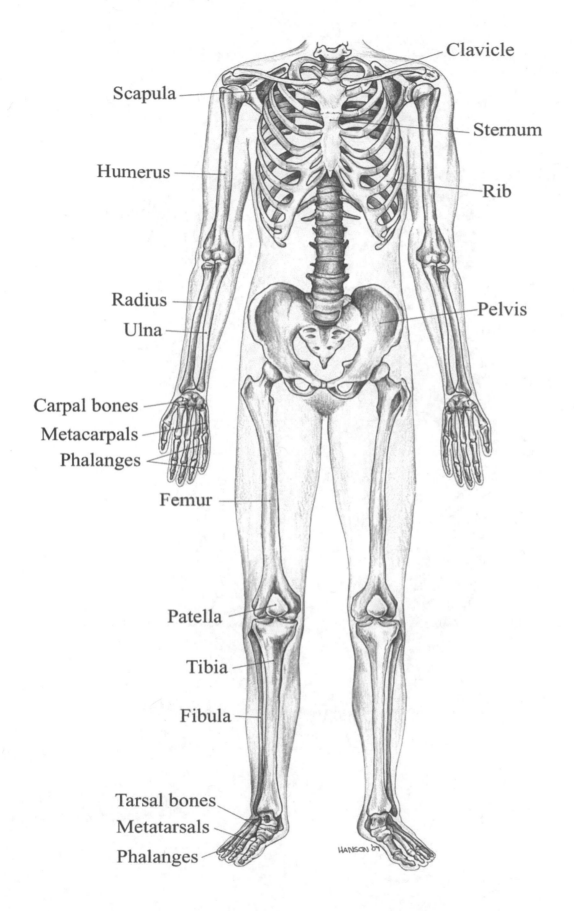

Clavicle

Scapula

Sternum

Humerus

Rib

Radius

Pelvis

Ulna

Carpal bones

Metacarpals

Phalanges

Femur

Patella

Tibia

Fibula

Tarsal bones

Metatarsals

Phalanges

HANSON 09

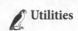

Cardiopulmonary Blood Flow

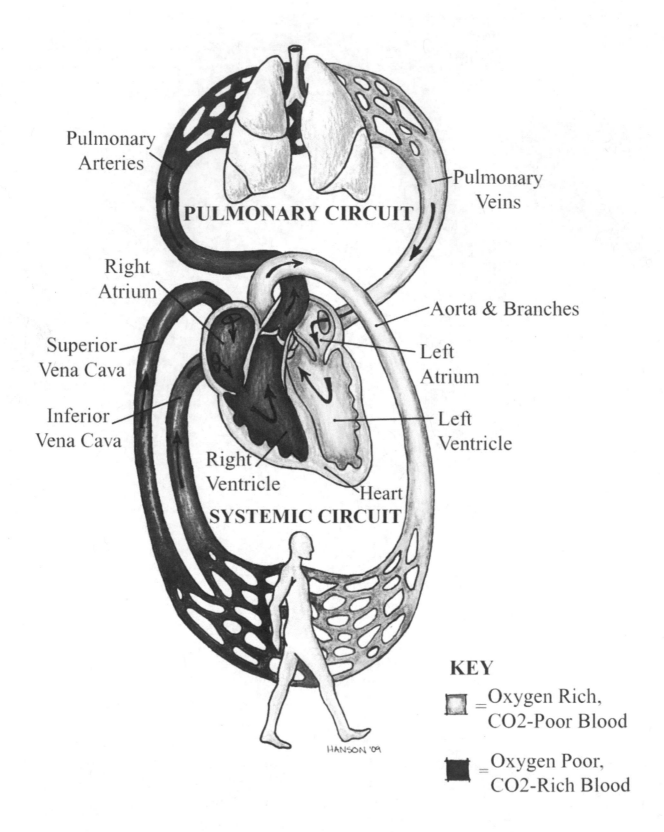

Pulmonary
Arteries

Pulmonary
Veins

PULMONARY CIRCUIT

Right
Atrium

Aorta & Branches

Superior
Vena Cava

Left
Atrium

Inferior
Vena Cava

Left
Ventricle

Right
Ventricle

Heart

SYSTEMIC CIRCUIT

HANSON '09

KEY

☐ = Oxygen Rich,
CO2-Poor Blood

■ = Oxygen Poor,
CO2-Rich Blood

Glossary

A

ABCDEs – Components of the Primary Survey: (massive hemorrhage), Airway, Breathing, Circulation, neurologic Deficit, and Environment.

ABD – Abbreviation for abdomen.

Acidosis - A condition caused by accumulation of acid or loss of base in the body.

Acute - Having rapid onset, severe symptoms, and a short course, not chronic.

Aerie – A raptor's nest; an elevated, often secluded location. We chose the name Aerie because of its connotations of wildness and the unique perspective gained in such a location.

Alveoli – Air sacs of the lungs where gas exchange occurs.

Ambulate – To walk- Ambulatory: able to walk

Anastomoses – Smaller arteries which form a link between main arteries.

Apnea - Absence of breathing.

Asphyxia - Suffocation.

Asystole – A lack of electrical activity in the heart seen as a flat line on electrocardiogram (ECG). Always associated with pulselessness and is not a shockable rhythm.

Aspiration - Drawing in or out as by suction. Foreign bodies may be aspirated into the nose, throat, or lungs on inspiration.

Auscultation - Listening for and interpreting sounds that occur within the body, usually with a stethoscope.

Avulsion – A flap of tissue that is not completely detached from the body

AVPU - Abbreviated neurological assessment scale - A=alert, V=verbal, P=pain, U=unresponsive.

B

BP - Blood Pressure, a vital sign; recorded as systolic blood pressure (SBP) over diastolic blood pressure (DBP) (e.g., 128/76). SBP is a measurement of pressure exerted against the walls of the arteries when the heart is contracted; DBP is a measurement of pressure exerted against the walls of the arteries when the heart is relaxed.

BSI - Body substance isolation.

C

Capillary Refill – The amount of time required for the capillaries to refill with blood after being compressed.

CNS - Central Nervous System (e.g., brain and spinal cord).

Conjunctivae – A thin clear moist membrane that coats the inner surfaces of the eyelids and the outer surface of the eye.

Convulsion - A violent, involuntary contraction or series of contractions of the voluntary muscles - a seizure.

CPR - Cardiopulmonary Resuscitation.

Crepitus - A grating sound heard and a sensation felt when the fractured ends of a bone rub together.

CSF - Cerebrospinal fluid - Fluid circulating around brain and spinal cord, cushioning brain and helping to remove by-products of brain metabolism. May leak out, particularly from ears and nose, with significant skull injuries.

CSM - Circulation, Sensation, and Motion or Motor function. Checked as part of the head to toe exam.

C-Spine - Cervical Spine. The uppermost 7 vertebrae of the spinal column.

Cyanosis – Bluish discoloration, observed first in the nail beds and oral mucosa, that results from inadequate oxygenation of the blood.

D

Dermatitis – Inflammation of the skin.

Diaphoresis - Profuse perspiration.

Distal - Farthest from center, from a medial line, or from the trunk.

Distended – Protruding beyond normal anatomic position, particularly used when referring to the abdomen and neck veins.

Dyspnea - Difficulty breathing.

E

Edema - The condition in which excess fluid

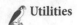

accumulates in body tissue, manifested by swelling.

Embolism - A mass (or *embolus*) of solid, liquid or gaseous material carried in the circulation which may lead to occlusion of blood vessels.

Epigastrium - The upper central portion of the abdomen within the sternal angle.

Epinephrine – Adrenalin. Hormone secreted by adrenal glands; used therapeutically as vasoconstrictor, cardiac stimulant, and to relax bronchioles. Its effects are brought about by stimulation of the sympathetic nervous system.

Erythema – Redness of the skin or mucous membrane.

Etiology - The causative agent of a disease or injury.

ETOH - Ethyl alcohol/ drinking alcohol.

Evisceration - To remove the intestines, to disembowel.

Exsanguinate - To bleed to death.

Extension - The movement by which both ends of any part are pulled part. A movement that brings the members of a limb into or toward a straight condition.

F

Febrile - Characterized by fever.

Flail Chest - The condition in which several ribs are broken, each in at least two places, or there is sternal fracture or separation of the ribs from the sternum, producing a free or floating segment of the chest wall.

Flexion - The act of bending.

Fx - Fracture.

G

GI Tract - Gastro-intestinal Tract.

Gangrene - Tissue death and decomposition from circulation obstructions or bacterial infections.

H

HEENT - Head, Eyes, Ears, Nose, and Throat.

Hemorrhagic - Related to abnormal internal or external discharge of blood. May be venous, arterial or capillary from blood vessels into tissues, into or from the body.

Hemothorax - Blood in the pleural cavity.

Herniation - Development of a hernia (protrusion or projection of an organ or a part of an organ through the wall of the cavity which normally contains it).

Hives – Also Urticaria. Often itchy, raised, red bumps on the skin often associated with allergic or anaphylactic reactions.

HR - Heart Rate. A vital sign.

Hx - History.

Hyperextension - Extreme or abnormal extension.

Hyperventilation - An increased rate and/or depth of respiration.

Hypoxia - Reduction of oxygen in body tissues below normal levels.

I

IC – Incident Commander (see Triage/ Multiple casualties)

ICP - Intracranial pressure. Increasing ICP is the primary cause of altered LOR in head injuries.

ICS – Incident Command System (see Triage).

Idiopathic – With no known cause.

Immunosuppressive – Lessening the ability for the immune system to function.

Integrity - The condition of being whole, not broken into parts.

Interstitial – Space or location between cells.

Intracellular - Within cells.

Intrathoracic – Within the thoracic (chest) cavity.

Ischemia – A decrease in blood supply to tissue resulting in inadequate oxygen delivery.

L

Lassitude – Weariness or lethargy.

Lethargy - Drowsiness or indifference.

LOR - Level of Responsiveness. A vital sign (see AVPU)

M

Malaise – Weakness and fatigue with vague discomfort.

MCI – Mass Casualty Incident

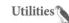

Medical Control - A process of medical oversight and quality control mechanisms implemented prior to, during, and after each medical event in an effort to ensure the highest possible level of patient care.

Melena – Dark black, tarry stools with a strong, characteristic odor; the result of partially digested blood from internal bleeding, typically from the upper digestive tract.

Mentation - Mental activity, often used in the context of describing a person's ability to think and reason.

Metabolism – The total of chemical reactions occurring in the cells of the body.

mmHg - Millimeters of Mercury

MOI - Mechanism of Injury.

N

NSAIDs – Non-Steroidal Anti-Inflammatory Drugs (see Medications).

N/V - Nausea and vomiting

Nasopharynx - Part of the pharynx situated above the soft palate.

Necrosis - Death of tissue, caused by loss of blood supply.

Neurological - Deals with the nervous system and its diseases.

Neurovascular - Concerning both the nervous and circulatory (vascular) systems.

O

Occlude – To obstruct or block an opening.

Occlusive Dressing - A watertight/airtight covering for a wound.

OPQRST - Used in patient questioning to elaborate on Signs/Symptoms.

Oropharynx - Central portion of the pharynx lying between the soft palate and upper portion of the epiglottis.

Oxygenation - Combination of oxygen with tissues of the body, happens when oxygen attaches to hemoglobin in the lungs. May also refer to oxygen saturation.

P

PWD - Abbreviation for skin, denoting Pink, Warm, Dry.

Palliate – To make feel better, to soothe.

Palpate - To examine by touch, to feel.

Paradoxical Movement - Abnormal movement of the chest wall in which inhalation causes a portion of chest wall to collapse; exhalation causes a segment to rise. See Flail Chest.

PERRL - An acronym for "Pupils Equally Round and Reactive to Light", represents normal pupil assessment.

Perfusion - Supplying an organ or tissue with nutrients and oxygen.

Peripheral - Located at, or pertaining to periphery; occurring away from the center.

Pharynx - Passageway for air from nasal cavity to larynx and food from mouth to esophagus.

Pneumonia – An infection of one or both lungs, typically from a bacterial or viral source.

Pneumothorax - Air in the pleural cavity or between the chest wall and lung.

Postictal State - The gradually resolving period of altered mentation and confusion after the convulsive state of a seizure that typically last 5 to 30 minutes.

Prone - Lying flat with the face downward.

Protocol - A written guideline outlining standards of care.

Proximal - Nearest point of attachment, center of the body, or point of reference. Opposite of distal.

Pt - Patient.

Pulmonary Edema - Accumulation of fluid in the alveoli that limits gas (carbon dioxide and oxygen) exchange between the blood and the airways.

R

Raccoon Eyes - Discoloration around both eyes, which may indicate basilar skull fracture.

RBCs - Red Blood Cells.

Rescue Breathing – A technique of providing artificial ventilations to a patient who is not breathing or not breathing adequately. Ventilations are delivered mouth-to-mouth, mouth-to-mask, or via bag-valve mask at a rate of 1 breath every 5 to 6 seconds.

Resuscitation - Restoring to life or consciousness, often using assisted breathing to restore ventilation and chest compressions/defibrillation to restore circulation.

RR - Respiratory Rate. A vital sign.

S

Sacrum – Lower portion of the spinal column, at the level of the pelvis.

SAMPLE - Used in patient questioning to identify potential causes of illnesses or problems, consisting of Signs/ Symptoms, Allergies, Medications, Past Medical History, Last Oral Intake, and Events.

Seizure – An abnormal electrical discharge in the brain causing an alteration in mental status with or without convulsive muscle activity.

SCTM - Abbreviation for skin color, temperature, moisture.

Shock - A state of inadequate tissue perfusion.

SMR - Spinal Motion Restriction.

SOAP Note - Documentation form for medical incidents.

Sputum - Mucus and other matter from the respiratory tract, usually coughed up.

Stabilization - To make stable or firm, to keep from changing.

Stridor - High-pitched sound typically heard on inspiration that is the result of upper airway constriction or obstruction.

Subcutaneous - beneath the skin.

Subluxation - Partial dislocation of a joint, so that the bone ends are misaligned but still in contact.

Supine - Lying flat with face upward.

Surfactant – Fluid found in the alveoli of the lungs.

Symmetry - Correspondence in shape, size, and relative position of parts on opposite sides of a body.

Sympathetic Nervous System - A division of the autonomic (involuntary) nervous system characterized by the "fight or flight" response which causes increased heart and respiratory rates and vasoconstriction.

Syncope – A transient loss of consciousness due to a lack of adequate blood flow to the brain; fainting.

T

Tachycardia - A rapid heart rate, over 100 per minute.

Tachypnea - Abnormally rapid respirations.

Tension Pneumothorax - A build up of pressure within the chest cavity, typically from air leaking out of an injured lung

Toxin - A poison.

Tracheal Deviation - A lateral shift in the position of trachea so it no longer appears in the mid-line of the neck.

Triage - A system used for categorization and sorting patients according to the severity of their problems.

Tx - Treatment.

U

Umbilicus - The belly-button.

Uvula - The extension of tissue at the back of the oral cavity that hangs above the throat.

V

Vasoconstriction - Constriction or narrowing of blood vessels.

Ventilatory - Related to ventilation of the lungs for purpose of oxygenation of blood.

Ventricular Fibrillation (V-Fib, VF) – The chaotic firing of cells in the ventricles of the heart seen as an erratic line on electrocardiogram (ECG). Always associated with pulselessness and is a shockable rhythm.

W

WEMT - Wilderness Emergency Medical Technician. A 200+ hour course, combining the traditional EMT curriculum and wilderness medicine topics.

WFA - Wilderness First Aid. A 16-hour wilderness medicine course.

WFR - Wilderness First Responder. A 72-hour wilderness medicine course.

Wheezing – High pitched, musical sound typically heard on expiration that is the result of constriction or obstruction of the lower airways in the lungs

WME – Wilderness Medicine Essentials. An 8-hour introductory course in wilderness medicine.

WMS - Wilderness Medical Society.